She Is Hit by Waves ...
But Will Not Sink

Paris' Battle with Neuroblastoma

Lauren Strickland

Published by BookLocker.com, Inc., Bradenton, Florida.

Printed in the United States of America on acid-free paper.

BookLocker.com, Inc.
2014

First Edition

Dedication

To my daughter Paris, who has been an example of extreme strength and has shaped our lives for the better, to our family and friends, and to the children fighting this disease today and those who will be unfairly chosen to fight tomorrow.

Acknowledgements

This story would not have been possible if it were not for the following very important people that have helped us along this journey. Without them I would have never been able to survive.

My daughter, Paris, who is the bravest, strongest person I know.

My husband, Ralph, for being a phenomenal father to our daughter. He is always loving and caring and never once saw her as anything but beautiful. As a husband, he has always been supportive and by my side through the roughest of times.

My entire family, especially my mother, Mary, step-father Tom and sister, Jennifer. Regardless of how much inconvenience it may have caused, no matter how much the cost, no matter how many sleepless nights, no matter how horrible the news, we all were ready to battle with everything we had and never gave up.

Individuals who have helped to make this book possible: Debra B. McCraw, freelance writer and editor; Veronica Hernandez with MAC makeup; Christy Weiss with Sunny Photography; Todd Engel with Engel Creative; and Booklocker Publishing.

Our friends and co-workers within District 200 and Joseph Academy who have supported us during this difficult journey.

Our extended families fighting neuroblastoma whom we have met along the way and the strangers who have entered our lives, showing us that we can handle any challenge that comes our way with endless support.

The educational staff of District 204: Ms. Allen, Mrs. Anderson, Mrs. Calkins, Mrs. Donovan, Ms. Hafer, Ms. Kalvaitis, Mrs. Rejniak, and

Ms. Schultz for being compassionate educators and ensuring that Paris receives the best educational experience possible.

Our friends at Northwestern Hospital in Chicago for their ongoing support for our family.

The local businesses, professional athletes, and teams that have donated to our fundraising efforts.

Our faith in God. We can't do anything but put it in his hands.

The Ronald McDonald House of New York City and volunteers for providing a home away from home.

Barbara Zobian, president of the New York Chapter of the Candlelighters Organization, and Rich Block, for ongoing support, providing an abundance of resources, and always going above and beyond for children and their families.

Midwest Miracle Mile Flights of Milwaukee, Steve Simon and Southwest Airlines, the staff of Corporate Angel Network, and Miracle Flights for providing medical transportation, making our out of state trips financially easier.

The Band of Parents organization and The Truth 365

And last but not least, our entire team, including volunteers, nurses, personal secretaries, social workers, physical therapists, nurse case managers, at-home nurse care providers, doctors, and surgeons at both Children's Memorial Hospital in Chicago and Memorial Sloan-Kettering in New York. In particular, I want to recognize Dr. Alden, Dr. Greyhack, Dr. Yasmin Gosiengfiao, Dr. Kramer, Dr. Kushner, Dr. LaQuaglia, Dr. Modak, Dr. Morrison, Dr. Reynolds, Dr. Waldon, Jacquie Toia, and Lisa Vanbokel who have worked so closely with our family throughout our journey thus far.

Table of Contents

Preface

My name is Lauren Strickland, and I am about to share my personal experience with neuroblastoma. My daughter, Paris, was diagnosed with the rare childhood cancer at just 9 days old. Yes, you read that correctly. I said 9 days old. I wanted to document my thoughts, feelings, and experiences so that the approximately 650 people whose children are diagnosed with neuroblastoma every year can see they are not alone in this journey and that at many times, others are feeling the exact same way. Should you find yourself on this journey, you may feel like at times you are going insane, as the road is rough. But if you look hard enough and maintain a hopeful spirit – and trust me, sometimes you have to dig really deep – good will come.

Before I begin this reflection process, I want to acknowledge all of the caretakers, whether you are the mothers, fathers, step-parents, aunts, uncles, guardians, or siblings who care for children with cancer. What we do is remarkable. There is no other job in the world like it, and it is by far the hardest, being physically, mentally, and emotionally exhausting. At times you feel like you just can't do it anymore, not for another second. But then you look at your child, and you gain an inner strength that makes you get up and continue on to the next day to face a new challenge. So for the times that you feel powerless, helpless, motionless, confused, depressed, sleep deprived, enraged, and like you can't continue, remember that you can.

After hearing our story, people are often first in shock and then in awe of how I have handled the situation as a mother. They proceed to tell me how strong I am, how they admire my strength and can't even begin to imagine what my life looks like. I truly appreciate those kind words. I often hear, "How do you handle it?"

My response is simple, "I do not have a choice – what else am I supposed to do?" I've realized that you don't know how much strength you have until being strong is the only choice you have.

I can't do anything but be strong. I can't sit around feeling sorry for myself and Paris, crying all of the time. I honestly don't have time to break down half as much as I would like too. Crying doesn't get the job done, and I have to fight to the end for Paris with all the strength that I wasn't even aware that I had. Sometimes I have to force myself to appear strong when I really don't feel any strength, but somehow I am able to manage and get through the day. Sometimes I begin to think I don't have it in me to break down; that I've built this permanent wall with limited emotions since I've been going strong for so long. I've almost forced myself to become emotionally immune to a certain degree.

When I do get a minute to myself, which is very rare, or when Paris' scans are stable and I have a moment to reflect on what life has dealt me, I allow myself to break down because I finally have time to process my emotions. If I were not in this situation and if I were looking in on someone else's life, I couldn't begin to understand or comprehend what they have to deal with on a daily basis.

In my eyes, Paris is the brave and courageous one. She is my best friend and my inspiration. She is really the driving force that keeps me going through all of the components of this unexpected outcome. Her determination, her overall demeanor, and her strong-willed character fit her perfectly. Of course there are times that I have thought to myself, this is too much to handle and that I can't fight for a single second longer – it's that emotionally and physically draining. But my quitting ultimately means giving up on Paris, which quickly puts things back into perspective. It's a fight for life. Even when she is suffering most, her little smile, loving stares, and unpredictable comments always amaze me. She is such a strong individual who has had to endure so much since the beginning of her life on Earth.

I am told that Paris is a hero, an inspiration, a role model. That she has so much strength, that she's a fighter. I admire that other people feel very passionately about Paris. She is just a little girl with no choice in this unfortunate matter, and since she has fought her whole life, she doesn't know any other way to be. She considers her trials and tribulations as simply part of her life.

My husband and I have to make difficult treatment decisions that result in countless unbearable and painful experiences, which could very well be classified as torture to the average person, in attempts to keep her alive. That's a hard pill for me to personally swallow, to consciously allow individuals to do horrendous things that one would never dream of, to my child, just to keep her alive. That took an emotional toll on me as a parent; it becomes mentally and physically exhausting and guilt driven, not to mention extremely stressful, but it's my reality and her way of life.

The lifestyle that we have encountered, I wish upon no one. The dynamic that I am living in is almost impossible to explain, but I'm going to try. Writing this book was personally therapeutic, and it allowed me to express my thoughts and feelings so that others may take what they see as valuable while they battle through the most unimaginable times. The book is also for Paris so that one day she can have a journal of the obstacles and constant battle that she fought every day to live.

As I analyze my story, I realize that I cross paths with people at certain times who have a lot of meaning to my life or that things that have happened in the past tend to resurface at my greatest times of need. I have met certain people at strange, unpredictable times that have happened to make the most thought-provoking comments right when I needed them. I found it helpful to listen to other families who shared their stories of neuroblastoma. The best advice that I can give is to remember that the only common bond is the word, "neuroblastoma." After that, every child is different. I hope that people take what they need, what's relevant or personal to them, after hearing my story and feel supported throughout this lifelong journey.

Everyone's experience with neuroblastoma is different, and there is no one way or right way. Everyone learns as they go, and they make decisions that sit well with them personally. What I chose to do others may be opposed to and vise versa. My goal is to provide you with as many resources, stories, and contact information as I can in an attempt to alleviate stress upon entering this "family." I remember when Paris was first diagnosed, I felt alone. I didn't even know what to ask or how to pronounce the medical terminology, but with time it came almost naturally and I began to feel as if it were second nature. I am hoping that this book gives you some guidance in a world that is very complicated, unknown, and scary, where fears are high and all we have is hope that binds us together.

Chapter 1: Wanting a Baby More Than Anything

I thought my life was perfect at 22. I had a lot of friends. I had finished college, earned multiple higher education degrees, and had an established career. I was living at home, saving all my money with no outstanding debt. I was single without any worries in the world.

My mother and my sister chose to be in the medical profession, but I was never interested in joining them. I honestly didn't know what I wanted to do, but as the time came for me to choose something, I chose teaching.

I found myself very interested in the field, truly feeling that I had the ability to teach individuals and provide an academic foundation as well as shape the lives of others who would go on to hopefully do great things within our society.

I finished the program in three years, taking every class available, and at times got permission to overload on classes. I obtained my undergraduate degree in special education and went on to obtain my English as a Second Language (ESL) endorsement. I then earned my masters in early childhood special education.

I wanted to start my life. I wanted to be an individual. I wanted to explore the world. At times, I think maybe I didn't take on this occupation subconsciously. Maybe I was destined to have this role to prepare me for what awaited me in my future.

In my early twenties, I had great expectations of what life would bring. In 2002 I toured my potential job site and ended up meeting my husband, whom I married in 2005. Ralph had three sons from previous relationships, and I was instantly placed into the role of a mother figure at 22. Yet, I never felt like I had the opportunity to be a mother on a full-time basis since the boys were only with us on the weekends.

There was just one thing missing from my life. I was 27 years old and wanted a baby more than anything. Many of my friends had children, so I was at the point in my life that I wanted that, too, and was financially and emotionally ready be a mother. Since 2006, every month my husband and I would look at pregnancy sticks, waiting the three minutes for them to reveal their answers, which seemed like forever. For a year, the sticks indicated "not pregnant."

It became a bit stressful as the months passed by. I thought about how people got pregnant after just one time, by mistake, or without even trying and how many are not initially pleased with the outcome. I analyzed that and thought to myself, "Wow, people are getting pregnant left and right who aren't even trying too, and people who are purposefully trying to get pregnant have to go through hell!"

My husband continuously told me, "It will happen when we're not expecting it to, and we can't plan this." Overall we balance each other very well, as he has a "half-full" positive personality, and I have a more "half-empty" perspective, or what I like to refer to as the realistic aspect of situations. By this point, I had spent so much money on countless brands of pregnancy tests, ovulation kits, and vitamins only to hear the grim news toward the end of each month. I was convinced it was not going to happen, but he continued to be hopeful.

I think back about that entire year that I was trying to conceive. Month after month, I never got pregnant. The same thing showed up on the pregnancy stick regardless of which way it was posed – the result was still no. I began to wonder if there was something wrong with me. How can I want something so badly and not get it? All around me people were pregnant, and I was starting to feel very disappointed.

In March 2007 I took yet another pregnancy test. I anticipated that it would be negative like all the others, but when I looked closer, I saw two lines. I was in shock, basically speechless. I couldn't remember

2

what the directions of the pregnancy test had stated, so I frantically re-read the information guide, which confirmed that I had finally become pregnant. I had planned out various ways to tell my husband in the event that I had gotten pregnant, however I was so ecstatic that I simply ran down the stairs and showed my husband the test screaming. That was one of the happiest moments in my life. I was going to be a mother to someone, a little life who I would care for and was prepared to be an excellent provider for.

Overall, my pregnancy was wonderful. I did everything right. I went to my routine doctor appointments, ate healthy, exercised, worked until the end of my pregnancy, read to the baby, spoke to the baby. I had no pains, no mood swings, and no cravings. Overall, I felt great! My doctor anticipated that I would gain between 25 and 30 pounds for the entire pregnancy; however I reached 25 pounds by month three. I gained a lot of weight over the nine months – about 67 pounds to be exact.

During one of final routine appointments, my OB/GYN began the discussion about labor and asked me if I wanted an epidural. I was positive that I did and asked her if she could make sure that she starred that area on the form so that no one would overlook it. I was so nervous about the final months and giving birth, as I had heard so many horror stories of excruciating pain and the problems that could arise. I couldn't even imagine the thought of pushing out a baby.

I got my first scare on June 27, 2007, when a routine ultrasound at 18 weeks 6 days, showed a 4 millimeter right choroid plexus cyst in the baby's brain. I remember my doctor explaining that typically these types of findings disappear over time but that she would like to schedule me for high-level ultrasounds from this point on. I had a million questions race through my mind. When you are pregnant, you just expect that things will be fine and your baby will be healthy. When you get news that states otherwise, you are put in a state of shock. All of my happiness just stopped, and being pregnant became very real. I now needed to deal with the fact that something could potentially be very wrong.

I could do nothing else but wait and worry. On July 19 and September 13, second and third high-level ultrasounds indicated that Paris was in a breech position and the area in question had subsided. I couldn't have been more relieved and thankful. I continued on with my pregnancy thinking Paris had a guardian angel watching over her. Little did we know this would be the first of many obstacles in Paris' life.

By the end of October, I could start to feel the uncomfortable effects of my pregnancy. I had developed carpal tunnel syndrome in my right hand, of course my writing hand. Then, exactly one week before Paris came; I developed Bell's palsy, which can cause a temporary facial paralysis. I woke up one morning and poured a glass of juice, and when I began to drink from the cup, it spilled everywhere. I noticed that I couldn't grasp my lip around the cup, causing the juice to spill onto my shirt and the floor. I ran to the mirror and noticed that I couldn't control the muscles on right side of my face, but I wasn't in pain.

I quickly called for Ralph, and he immediately thought I was having a mild stroke. We went to the hospital, and the doctor assessed my condition. She asked me if I could blow out my cheeks. I attempted to demonstrate the task and proceeded to try. I thought I could, but only the left side of my face responded. She confirmed that I couldn't demonstrate the task when I tried it in front of the mirror. There was not much she could do other than prescribe steroids for it.

I was due with Paris in seven days, so I dealt with the Bell's palsy. Ralph humored himself as he joked with my appearance. I was unable to chew food or smile. I drooled constantly. I couldn't formulate my words or speak correctly. I couldn't even close my right eye, so sleeping was extremely difficult. I suffered from Bell's palsy for a total of three months. All of my labor and delivery pictures with Paris looked horrible.

My last regular OB/GYN appointment was scheduled for November 20. Paris was due on November 22, which was Thanksgiving Day. My appointment was at 4 p.m., and I packed an overnight bag assuring Ralph that I was not coming home without having the baby. Ralph and I drove to the appointment, and overall I felt great. While in the waiting room, I felt abdominal pain like I had never felt before. The doctor examined me and confirmed that I was having timed contractions. They got stronger by the second, and I immediately was monitored for a few hours. My 4 p.m. appointment continued until 6:30. My doctor gave me the choice – to either go home and be admitted the following day or to be admitted later on that night once I went home and gathered my things. I was one step ahead and already had a packed bag with me, so Ralph and I chose to be admitted.

The pain was very intense. The team checked me in, and I was finally settled into a room. At this point, my family had arrived. At 3 centimeters the doctors broke my water, and I felt a combination of the most excruciating pain and relief. I was given so much pain medicine that I don't remember much. The medication caused me to break out in red patches all over my body, especially my face. My nose was bright red and severely itched. My younger sister saw this as prime opportunity to video tape me mumbling, rambling, and scratching the inside of my nose with the end of a plastic spoon.

By 9 p.m. I was not dilating past 3 centimeters and Paris' heart rate was severely dropping with every contraction. The team decided immediately to do a Cesarean. In an instant, everything changed. All I remember was being pushed into a bright room with many people wearing blue sterile suits. I remember seeing my husband for a second holding a sterile gown as I rolled by him, and then all I remember was that it was just the doctor and I alone in a brightly lit room. She was preparing me for the long-awaited epidural. She asked me to sit up and hold onto her and not to move. I held onto her, and in an instant the pinch was over. It was simple. Literally, it felt like a little pinch. I would recommend an epidural to anyone in a heartbeat without the painful description.

The next thing I remember is my legs became so heavy and I couldn't lift them at all even though I tried very hard and used all of my might. My last memory was hearing the doctor say to someone, "Pass scalpel number nine." I couldn't remember the rest of the process if I tried – I had completely blacked out.

When I awoke, I caught a glimpse of Ralph to my side. He was not present for the surgery, but the team let him into the sterile room after it was over. He witnessed them stapling me up, and then he tended to the baby, cutting the remains of her umbilical cord. He told me that I did a great job, and then I fell back into a state of unconsciousness.

Twenty-six minutes from the time they took me away, I awoke in the original delivery room where everyone was gathered to see our new baby, Paris. She was born Tuesday, November 20, 2007, at 9:26 p.m., weighing 7 pounds and 13 ounces.

I saw how beautiful she was. Most importantly, she was declared healthy. The little girl that I had hoped for and wanted for so long was finally here looking at me right in the eyes. I thought to myself as I held her, "I will be responsible for this little person for the rest of my life." As I held her, there became an unspoken bond between us. I knew I would do anything for her to keep her safe and do everything that a mother should do for her child. At that moment, I became second and Paris became first.

I was discharged from the hospital on Saturday, November 24, 2007, and looked forward to bringing my new baby home and welcoming her into the world. I looked forward to being at home with her for the duration of my three-month maternity leave. Little did I know my lifelong commitment and dedication to our daughter was going to start very quickly.

Chapter 2: From Normal to Abnormal

I vividly remember telling my principal that I was pregnant and would only be taking the allowed three months of maternity leave. I also told him that I had plans to finish my administrative certificate and that I was a woman who wanted to have a baby but also wanted to work. He quickly responded, "Once you see that baby, you won't come back. Should I look for someone else? I have a feeling that you won't be coming back."

I responded, "I'll be back. Just wait and see."

I had every intention to returning to work after my leave had ended. I worked very hard to get where I was and had plans on taking my career further. My leave chose me; I didn't choose to stop working for the year to take care of Paris. I missed my co-workers and the routine of a normal day. I had become a stay-at-home mother, which also had its benefits because I was able to spend every minute with Paris, watching her grow. I was solely responsible, impacting her growth and development every step of the way.

At 9 days old my whole agenda had changed. Not one thing that I had planned for had remained the same, and I had to plan all over again for something bigger.

On November 26, 2007, six days after Paris was born, we noticed that her abdomen was extremely distended to the right. Ralph and I took her to our local hospital where her pediatrician was established and immediately questioned the distended area. She examined Paris' abdomen and found it to be within normal limits. The medical notes specifically state that the distention was considered normal and was related to Paris being "full," as we had reported that she just ate. The pediatrician attributed it to gas. When she dismissed our concern as being nothing out of the ordinary, we didn't question it and went home. She assured me that I was a new young parent and that it was nothing to be concerned about and reiterated that Paris was healthy.

After three days, her abdomen was still distended and did not look as if it decreased in size. We were concerned, as it certainly did not resemble an infant being full or having gas. It literally looked as if my six-day-old baby was nine months pregnant. No one can fathom the description of her abdomen until they actually see the picture. Once they do, they are in complete shock.

On November 29, my mother and her friend came over to my house to help watch Paris, allowing me to get some much-needed rest. Both my mother and her friend are in the medical profession, and when they arrived, I told them about Paris' abdomen and our visit with the pediatrician. I asked my mother to confirm what I saw, and upon first glance she, too, was very concerned and instructed me to call our pediatrician back right away and request to be seen that day. The first available opening was at 4 p.m.

My mother and her friend instructed me to take a nap before our appointment, as I was sleep deprived, and assured me that they would take care of Paris. As a new mom, I personally battled with having someone else watch Paris, but I knew I needed some rest and still didn't feel 100 percent. As I went upstairs to lie down, I just couldn't fall asleep. I felt this push to force myself to stay awake and check on Paris to make sure she was alright. I didn't end up napping that day but instead talked with our visitors about my concerns with Paris. I suppose my "mother's instinct" knew that something was wrong.

I remember calling my husband to inform him that Paris' abdomen had not decreased in size and we were going to the pediatrician again to assess the situation. He was concerned and wanted to leave work early to meet me at the appointment, but I assured him not to worry and said, "There's no emergency. We think everything is fine, but we were going anyway."

I asked him to meet me there after work. My mother and stepfather accompanied me to the appointment at 4:00 p.m. As we waited in the waiting room, a part of me began to worry. I began to think the worst, as her abdomen hadn't resolved itself in three days. I began to question what if something was wrong but quickly adjusted my way of thinking, verbally reassuring myself by saying, "What could really be wrong, the pediatrician said she's healthy." I think at that point I was teeter-tottering with the realization that something very well could be wrong, I just didn't know what it was so I was trying to convince myself that it was really nothing.

I was called into the office where the pediatrician again examined Paris. She noticed and examined the same distended area that I brought to her attention three days prior. Her facial expression now seemed more concerned, as I think she herself thought that it would have resolved itself. I remember sitting in the office and my mother questioning if the area could be a mass of some sort and insisted that we were not leaving until further imaging was done to rule out the possibility of a mass.

This time, the pediatrician noted in her report that there was "an asymmetric bulge in the right upper quadrant, positive palpable soft mass, does not feel hard like liver." She also examined her back indicating that "right thoracic area positive for lump with vascular pattern under skin, firm non-mobile, not tender." She noticed and noted that Paris had some twitching of the right lower extremity. Comparing these observations to those from our last appointment, the diagnosis of Paris' back and abdomen changed from normal to abnormal. The pediatrician documented in the additional note section that there is a sudden growth of a right-upper-quadrant abdominal mass and a right-back lump. She wanted to rule out tumor versus cyst, hydronephrosis versus ovarian pathology, but given the combination of symptoms, she needed to rule out neuroblastoma versus Wilms tumor versus leukemia, which she doubted. After the examination and now alarming concern, the pediatrician advised us that we take Paris to the emergency room for lab work, an ultrasound, and further imagining.

My mom, stepfather and now Ralph arrived in the waiting room of the emergency room and waited and waited. At this point, I was in a complete daze. I remember holding Paris and rocking her, cuddling her, and crying hysterically. An ultrasound tech took Paris. The imagining took an extremely long time, so my mother and I demanded to see where Paris was and sit with her during the imagining. Another tech brought us into the room. My mother saw a mass on the image. She questioned the tech, and he said he hadn't seen anything like that before. Then he left the room and said he needed to consult with another tech and never returned.

As we were waiting in the ultrasound room, I remember asking my mom, "What does that mean, Mom, what does that mean?"

My mom responded, "I think she has cancer, and I think it's very bad." Now my hysteria has just become worse. We returned to the waiting room with complete confusion and shock. They kept Paris to perform a CT scan. Again, we were in the waiting room for an extremely long time. After reflecting on the incident, I think that it took so long because they didn't sedate Paris and had to take multiple images. We sat in the waiting room from 4:30 until 10:30 p.m., my emotions ranged from panic to hysteria. I remember making one phone call in particular to my friend that I worked with. All I remember is calling her crying, saying, "Yolanda, I'm at the hospital with Paris." I asked her to please pray for my baby.

In all honestly I was in complete shock and can't vividly remember the events of that night clearly. Cancer, Cancer, Cancer ... what did she have? What were these words that sounded so foreign to me? I knew what they were but couldn't piece the puzzle together. I feel like I was in a trance, not remembering anything clearly. I remember tidbits, and it is so difficult even now to put the pieces together to retell a coherent story of that evening. I remember rocking back and forth. I remember feeling blank. At some points, it seemed like everything was moving around me quickly and I couldn't move. At other times, it felt like everything was moving in slow motion. I remember chanting at one point, repeating "What's wrong with my baby?" over and over. I don't remember anyone speaking. I can only place myself sitting in the waiting room in the chair second to the left.

I received another phone call from the doctor to confirm that Paris had a mass, and the world stopped. Somehow, we moved from the waiting room and someone brought us into a holding room, I assume because the imaging area was closing for the night. The doctor and our pediatrician arrived at some point, and I vividly remember them telling us that it greatly appears to be neuroblastoma, but there's a chance that it could be a Wilms tumor.

As I was gathering our things and walking out, I remember someone making a comment in passing that I better pray that it is a Wilms tumor and not neuroblastoma.

The doctor discussed the results of the ultrasound and CT scan. The ultrasound of the abdomen showed a soft tissue mass adjacent to the spine. That report was followed by a CT scan of the chest, abdomen, and pelvis, which showed a mass that measured 7.4 by 2.9 by 4.1 centimeters. It spanned from the T7 to T12 vertebral bodies with intraspinal extension, placing Paris at risk for spinal cord compression. The mass extended to the nerve root foramen of T8, T9, and T10. The extension of the tumor surrounded the inferior vena cava and straddled the right hemidiaphragm. It destroyed her seventh and eighth ribs. An emergent MRI confirmed spine compression and the primary thoracic neuroblastoma.

I believe that those traumatic words permanently caused me to shut down, and my coping strategy was to blank out everything after I heard them. I looked around, and all of a sudden I saw my mom, stepfather and Ralph – the look of fear and disbelief that appeared instantaneously on their faces are permanently engraved in my mind.

Their faces indicated that something horrific was about to happen. I immediately got the impression that she was going to die. Images flashed through my mind. I just met Paris nine days ago, and now someone was telling me that there was a chance she was critically ill with cancer that had the potential to kill her. We were instructed to go straight to Children's Memorial Hospital in Chicago, as Rush was not specialized in working with children.

From this point on, my recollection of events are in disarray or non-existent. The entire situation and information that I had just been given literally put me into a state of shock. Somehow I got in the car. Everything was moving in slow motion around me. I remember hearing people talking, but it all sounded like muttering. I can't recall any part of the conversation for the entire 45-minute drive from Aurora to Children's Memorial Hospital, located in downtown Chicago. The only thing I remember is sitting next to Paris, all bundled up in her snowsuit, wide awake with her big brown eyes staring at me the entire way. Everything else felt black around me as if everyone else did not exist. I remember resting my head on her as we drove. Everything in my mind was empty, blank and dark. I felt helpless, and the next thing I remember is pulling into the emergency room area at the hospital. I felt like I wasn't in control of my mind. I was just going through motions, and somehow they were correct, but I can't recall them to this day.

When we arrived at Children's Memorial Hospital, the emergency team was waiting for us. My sister had arrived and was waiting for us as well. At this point, it was well past 11 p.m. From that point forward, everything happened so quickly. The oncology team decided to do an MRI on Paris to determine how severe the tumor was. By the time we got settled in a room and I glanced at the time, it was past 1 a.m. On November 29, we began our inpatient stay at Children's Memorial Hospital, where we would remain until December 12.

Chapter 3: Welcome to the Cancer World

"I know it seems like an immovable mountain, but it is not. Step by step you will climb until suddenly without warning you will see how far you have come." – Jess, taken from an excerpt from a diary of a mom

In life when you're not faced with a situation, you believe in your mind that the unthinkable is impossible to handle. But when you're actually in that "unthinkable" situation, it's amazing how you can obtain inner strength to handle and deal with situations that you never fathomed. You didn't choose this…it chose you…so you need to choose to fight.

I went from being a regular, hard-working, middle-class person to in an instant being thrown into a situation that no one is ever prepared for. My background is in education and administration, however after all of this I received a crash course in medicine. Sometimes I think to myself, if I would have had a little insight into the future, I would have went right into medicine rather than dedicating my whole life to my educational career.

I remember them telling me that Paris has neuroblastoma. I couldn't even repeat the word, it sounded so foreign to me. I remember having to ask, "She has what again? Can you spell it? What did you say? She has what? Can you say it slowly? What does that even mean?" Now, not only do I use the word neuroblastoma frequently, but I know it along with countless other medical terms that I never thought would be in my vocabulary. People around me are amazed when I speak to doctors or medical professionals about her condition.

Prior to us receiving the news that Paris was diagnosed with cancer, we never had exposure to children with cancer. I never thought of childhood cancer even though I saw the faces of it on television through advertisements for hospitals. I always thought that cancer was horrific but ultimately became disconnected with the concept, as so many people do unless they are directly affected. Now I was directly affected. I had to battle every day just to give my daughter a fighting chance at surviving this horrific disease.

"Life doesn't care about your vision," from the movie "Knocked Up," was probably one of the best quotes that I ever heard. I sit and think about how we have all envisioned our life to be. One of the hardest things to do is to accept change. Facing the realization and coming to terms that regardless of how I thought it was going to be, this is what it is and this is how now it's not.

Now I'm a cancer mom. Sometimes I wish I was just a "normal" mother. I often say, I just want to be a mom. I don't want to be bombarded with the medical terminology. I don't want to have to remember everything – dates, appointments, returning calls, treatment plans, side effects, long-term effects that are still unpredictable, paperwork from insurance and ongoing hospital bills. Sometimes I wonder, how did I get here, how did this happen or why did I get chosen for this role? In the past, I worried about other minimal everyday life things, never cancer in children.

Once you're a cancer mom, your world changes. Nothing is trivial, and nothing is seen as minor. I tend to overreact about everything because unfortunately our worst fear of "it's nothing, your child is healthy," turned into a rush to the emergency room with a diagnosis of cancer in a seven-hour timeframe. Our life has forced us to look at the world differently, in a way that I never thought that I would. My eyes seem to be more focused on what really matters in life.

The infamous question that everyone dealing with cancer asks themselves at one point or another is why? I ponder why Paris, an innocent child, not being able to experience truly the first two years, was prisoner in a hospital. Why was it her to be one of the children chosen to go through this? Realistically, I will never know the reason or answer. The equation doesn't make sense to me. It never will. In reality, the real question should be why anyone – especially children who haven't even begun their lives.

Every three-and-a-half minutes a child is diagnosed with cancer. Within a four-hour span, 69 children will be newly diagnosed and their parents will hear the devastating words, "Your child has cancer." Every four hours, a child with cancer dies. It's difficult not to allow your mind to become stuck on the concept of why. There were 649 other parents in 2007 asking the same question who heard the same words, and there were 649 children who dealt and continue to deal with having cancer.

I kept thinking about my pregnancy and what I did, trying to evaluate it. Questioning what I ate, where I went, or what prenatal vitamin I took because I switched it about three times. Did that have something to do with it? I made all of my appointments; I exercised but gained a lot of weight. I questioned everything.

There seem to be many autoimmune issues among families who have children with neuroblastoma, such as hyperthyroidism – overactive tissue in the thyroid gland – and hypothyroidism – underactive thyroid that is not producing an adequate amount of the thyroid hormone.

Many women with children who have neuroblastoma were diagnosed with gestational diabetes during pregnancy or soon afterward. Many women also have breast cancer, and many children who are diagnosed were born with hemangiomas (strawberry birthmarks). Paris had one at birth on her left hand, between her middle and ring finger.

I think about pesticides and insect bites. We commonly use pesticides on our lawn. My husband is an avid golfer and on treated lawns on a regular basis. Homes built prior to 1988 may have pesticide-treated lumber to prevent termites.

Whenever I met someone whose child also had neuroblastoma, we tried to identify some commonality among us. You feel like if you don't think about everything or if you don't throw it out there for others to compare to, you may be missing the common thread. But after awhile it makes you crazy. You can stop and analyze it forever, but to this day there is no rhyme or reason. It just is.

The truth is, there is no answer, which I believe is one of the most difficult things to come to terms with. I sometimes think that if I at least had a reason to why this occurred, I may be able to process this entire thing better. The cycle continues, and new families are exposed to this cancer world every year. I have to keep reminding myself if I continue to be stuck in the "Why?" state of mind, I can't move forward and take care of Paris to the best of my ability. I've had to force myself to find the positive in all the bad. I have had to dig really deep sometimes to find the positive angle on things because the negative is very obvious and the positive seems to be always buried. Sometimes "why" is unanswerable, which is unfortunate because we all feel like we need answers to the unknown. When you accept your role as being special and unique and despite that you are an undoubtedly excellent caretaker, it's inevitable to think about how the hand that you got dealt is very unfair.

It's surprising how many families are going through the same thing, just hidden within the "normal" population. Disease is a horrible thing in itself. However, if you examine it closely, it can also be viewed as a positive thing because it strangely bridges the gap between people. I once heard, "Healing doesn't mean the elimination of the illness, but it could mean that the person or people around it are being transformed because of it." Parents living through the dynamic of cancer live by hope. Hope is the driving force that keeps us going. With hope comes strength.

There are countless individuals who have perfectly healthy children and do not see the value in what they have been blessed with. There are so many parents who don't take the time to communicate with them, care for them, provide their basic needs, interact with them, provide them with exploratory experiences, read with them, do school work with them. It's just not happening. I think to myself, if children with parents like that can't find the time to participate in the basic needs of children, then what would they do with a child who is chronically sick? That's where Ralph reminds me that this is why we are Paris' parents.

"Each choice we make causes a ripple effect in our lives. When things happen to us, it is the reaction we choose that can create the difference between the sorrows of our past and the joy of our future."
– Chelle Thompson, editor of Inspiration Line

Chapter 4: Neuroblastoma

Think about this for a minute … the average human male ejaculate contains 50 to 500 million sperm cells. I was really shocked when I learned this. I actually had good reason now to think about it. Out of all of the possible sperm cells present, one out of the 50 million happened to be my daughter Paris, who happened to be diagnosed with cancer. Was it just destined to be that way? I pondered whether we would be faced with the same situation if we conceived the night before, the night after, the month before, the month after. Out of all of those sperm cells … that one that was claimed as Paris had a complication.

Sometimes I think I was chosen for this role. I was established in my life and married. I was certainly prepared. I had a career that provided me with health care, and I am the type of person that if you tell me I can't, I will prove that I can. I think about all of those millions of sperm cells that could have been fertilized. Why did Paris get chosen? Why did hers have to be the one that was going to be sick? All of these questions lead me to think that I was supposed to get pregnant at that particular time, Paris was supposed to enter this world, and I was supposed to take care of her no matter what. I believe that Paris is here for a very important reason, as all other children battling cancer or any other life-threatening illness are, too, making them all very special children.

As Paris began more and more treatment and her chances of overall survival lessened, I began to wonder about all of the milestones and firsts that parents typically share with their child. The first roll, the first yawn, the first real laugh, the first crawl, the first step, the first words; especially hearing, "I love you," experiencing potty training, scheduling play dates, doing crafts, experiencing mommy and daughter interactions, painting finger and toe nails, doing hair, planning birthdays, hearing the first joke, knowing your child's likes and dislikes, the first zoo trip, wiggling her first tooth and watching the excitement of the tooth fairy taking it away, preparing for Santa, listening to her made-up songs and imaginative play, listening to her first problem and helping her solve it, rewarding her for doing something great, coming to her aide when she falls down and gets hurt, watching her pick out her mismatched clothes, the first day of kindergarten, answering the infamous question of why, listening to her read her first story all by herself, watching her ride a bike, having her help me bake or cook. Then watching her attending high school, teaching her about being confident, teaching her life lessons, learning her personality, driving, dating, proms, graduation, choosing a career, planning a wedding; all of those things that parents long to be a part of.

I envisioned witnessing some of these milestones over the first three months of my maternity leave and throughout a lifetime in the comfort of my home. I never thought that I would have to witness many of them from a hospital room or even wonder if she would reach the milestones that I had hoped to witness. Fear began to consume me, and I questioned the possibility that I may never witness these things, as the chances of my daughter's survival were in great jeopardy due to the realistic fact that her illness had the potential to take her life away.

Paris was officially diagnosed with neuroblastoma, a childhood cancer that affects approximately 650 children, typically between the ages of 2 and 5 years old, each year worldwide. Out of those 650 kids, 50 are under the age of 1. Paris was 1 out of those 49 children worldwide.

When Paris was first diagnosed, I couldn't tell you a thing about it let alone how to say it correctly. Now, six years later, I can tell you everything there is to know – what hospitals are considered the best, what treatment plans are out there, what organizations are dedicated to the disease. I have become an expert in a field that no one should even have to experience. The only thing I can't tell you about neuroblastoma is what causes it and how to cure it. My one wish in life is to be able to tell you. Trust me, I am dying to know. Someone out there has the answer – it is just waiting to be discovered. The cure is under our fingertips. Advances in technology and medicine have come such a long way, and one day, without a doubt, we will find the cure that we are all waiting for.

Neuroblastoma is a horrific childhood cancer that develops from nerve cells and typically affects the central nervous system. Neuro refers to nerves and blastoma refers to a cancer that affects immature or developing cells. Neurons are the main component of the brain and spinal cord, and nerves that connect them to the rest of the body. During its development, a fetus makes immature nerve cells known as neuroblasts, which eventually turn into nerve cells and fibers and the cells that make up the adrenal gland. The majority of them mature at birth and eventually disappear.

The thought is that malignant tumors called neuroblastoma occur when normal fetal neuroblasts fail to become mature nerve cells. Instead, they continue to grow and divide. Studies have shown that small clusters of neuroblasts are common in infants younger than 3 months old; however, they often mature into nerve tissue or disappear. Sometimes they remain, and as they continue to grow, they form tumors that can spread to other parts of the body, commonly the abdomen. Neuroblastoma is the most common extracrainal (outside of the brain) solid tumor in children.

Most neuroblastoma cases involve abnormalities – either a deletion or rearrangement – to chromosome 1, which causes amplification or multiple copies of the oncogene MYCN. Oncogenes are genes that promote uncontrolled cell division. Chromosome 1, considered to be the largest human chromosome, spans 247 million DNA building blocks and represents 8 percent of the total DNA in cells. In 2004, a group of German researchers reported that a series of neuroblastomas demonstrated a consistent pattern of deletions and over-representations on chromosomes 3, 10, 17q, and 20. Studies of localized tumors were characterized by the loss of the whole chromosomes 3, 4, 10, and 16 and gains of 6, 7, 8, 13, 17, 18, and 20.

When genes are deleted on a particular section of chromosome 11, the result is aggressive neuroblastoma. Studies have shown that children tend to have a decreased overall survival rate when there is a higher level of MYCN and when there is a 1P or 11Q loss and 17Q gain. The suppressor gene called TrkA is considered biologically favorable; however, the TrkB expressing tumors that have MYCN amplification are aggressive and often fatal.

It has recently been determined that neuroblastoma originates due to a mutated gene identified as the ALK gene, although the exact cause is currently unknown. Each time a cell divides, it must copy approximately 6,000 million letters of the DNA code. Most errors are corrected immediately, but a few manage to escape unnoticed. Occasionally gene mutation can occur at any point in one's life when a cell makes errors in copying its genes. Mutations in certain crucial genes can cause abnormal cell growth and eventually turn a healthy cell into a cancerous one.

Oncologists who specialize in the field of neuroblastoma classify the disease through stages and risk groups.

The International Neuroblastoma Staging System (INSS) has five stages:

- Stage 1 indicates that the tumor is localized, has not crossed the midline of the body, and hasn't metastasized, or spread. All of the visible tumor can be completely removed with surgery. When examined under the microscope, the tumors edges may contain tumor cells. Lymph nodes enclosed within the tumor cells may contain tumor cells, but lymph nodes outside the tumor cell are cancer free.

- Stage 2 indicates that the tumor is localized but because of its size, location, or relationship to other organs, most of it can be removed with surgery. It is still only located on one side of the body. As with Stage 1, lymph nodes enclosed within the tumor cells may contain tumor cells, but lymph nodes outside the tumor cell are cancer free.

- Stage 3 is considered advanced and indicates that the cancer cannot be removed with surgery alone. It has crossed the midline (defined as the spine) to the other side of the body. It may or may not have spread to the lymph nodes. It may have originated on one side of the body and metastasized to nearby lymph nodes on the other side of the body or it is located in the middle of the body and growing toward both sides.

- Stage 4 is considered advanced, meaning the cancer has metastasized to other parts of the body, such as the lymph nodes, bones, liver, skin, bone marrow, and/or other organs.

- Stage 4S is considered a special category of neuroblastoma and applies to children who are younger than 1 year. The cancer is on one side of the body and is localized. It may have spread to lymph nodes on one side of the body but not to those on the opposite side. The neuroblastoma has spread to the skin, liver, and/or bone marrow. Neuroblastoma at this stage sometimes goes away on its own and may not require treatment.

Neuroblastoma is also categorized into four risk groups:

- Low risk includes all children who are stage 1; any child who is stage 2 and younger than 1 year old; any child who is stage 2 and older than 1 year but is MYNC non-amplified; any child who is stage 2, older than 1 year and is MYNC amplified but has a favorable histology; and any child who is stage 4S with a favorable histology and is hyperdiploid and MYNC non-amplified.

- Intermediate risk includes any child who is stage 3, younger than 1 year and MYNC non-amplified; any child who is stage 3, older than 1 year, MYNC non-amplified and has a favorable histology; any child who is stage 4, younger than 1 year and MYNC non-amplified; and any child who is stage 4S, younger than 1 year, MYNC non-amplified and has normal DNA ploidy or unfavorable histology.

- High risk is defined as any child who is stage 2, older than 1 year and MYNC amplified and has an unfavorable histology; any child who is stage 3, younger than 1 year and MYNC amplified; any child who is stage 3, older than 1 year, and MYNC non-amplified and has an unfavorable histology; any child who is stage 3, older than 1 year and MYNC amplified; any child who is stage 4, younger than 1 year and MYNC amplified; any child who is stage 4 and older than 1 year; and any child who is stage 4S, younger than 1 year and MYNC amplified.

- Ganglioneuroblastoma Nodular, a rare subtype containing immature nerve cells, is classified as high risk. This intermediate tumor contains both malignant (fast-growing and likely to spread) and benign (slow-growing and unlikely to spread) cells. It can either grow abnormally, or it can mature and stop dividing, causing the tumor to be classified as ganglioneuroma, which is benign.

Neuroblastoma does not discriminate. It has the potential to affect infants, children, and at times teenagers or adults differently, in all different places within the body. It has the potential to attack any age group, race, gender, religion, age, or socioeconomic class of people and in any location, worldwide. To give a prognosis is very difficult because each child responds to treatment differently, tolerates it differently, and has different side effects. It carries itself differently in each person. There is no noted common thread between any one person and neuroblastoma. There may be similarities among people, but no case is exactly alike. Doctors use treatment plans as a guide but often tailor them to fit the specific needs of the child. It's like trying to find someone in the world with exactly the same fingerprint.

Chapter 5: Our Journey Begins

December 1, 2007

The team discussed our religious beliefs with us and advised that if we wanted to have Paris baptized that we perform it immediately, as they believed her little body may not be able to tolerate the intense toxic chemotherapy that she would soon endure. Just imagine getting this news. We agreed for Paris to be baptized at the hospital, which is considered the sacrament. Although you can participate in the baptismal ceremony again later in a church, the child would only be truly baptized once, and that is in the hospital. We decided do this, without a white gown, extended family or friends, and without celebration of her life. We were baptizing her in a plea to God to allow her to remain on Earth and watch over her through this horrific situation. The chaplain came into our hospital room and baptized Paris with Ralph and I feeling and looking like pure shit, crying at the thought that we were baptizing her because we thought we might lose her. Her godfather is a stranger, a bystander from the hospital who we don't even know. I am very thankful that my sister was there to sign the certificate as Paris' godmother.

Every inpatient roommate Paris had in Chicago and New York, as well as the people with whom we have crossed paths along this journey, have taught us something along the way. Our first roommates, Ellen and her daughter Kelly, at Children's was no exception. Ellen had been down this road many times before with Kelly, who had been diagnosed with medulloblastoma at only 4 years old. I honestly couldn't have been paired with a more appropriate roommate that night. Ellen was calm, probably after years of practice, realistic, tough, and positive all at the same time. Looking back, she taught me a lot of life lessons and gave me valuable advice during those first couple of inpatient days. She also gave me a crash course on the days to come, preparing me for my future.

We began our treatment plan at 10 days old. Early on the morning of December 2, 2007, Paris underwent a biopsy of the thoracic area, specifically T9 and T10. Biopsies require a sample of the tumor to be taken. The doctor removes the sample and examines it under a microscope to find any cells that may be cancerous. It is said that neuroblastoma cells tend to be blue in color.

Later that day, the doctors placed a broviac/central line for Paris to receive chemotherapy and medications. This catheter is passed through the vein to end up in the chest (thoracic) portion of the large vein returning blood to the heart (vena cava) or in the atrium of the heart. Between December 2, 2007, and January 30, 2008, Paris endured four cycles of Carboplatin, Etoposide (VP16), Cytoxan, and Doxorubicin through a central line rather than undergoing surgery to remove the tumor. Initially, surgery was too risky of an option because the tumor was compressing her spinal cord. The chemotherapy regiment was on an outpatient basis. We would arrive at the hospital early in the morning, and Paris would receive ondansetron, a medication to prevent nausea and vomiting, before starting her scheduled chemotherapy. We were then able to take her home in the evening rather than spending the night in the hospital. Paris also received an oral antibiotic of co-trimoxazole/trimethoprim-sulfa for three consecutive days each week for the duration of treatment to prevent pneumonia.

Chemotherapy treatments commonly used to treat neuroblastoma include cyclophosphamide or ifosfamide, cisplatin or carboplatin, vincristine, doxorubicin, etoposide, teniposide, and topotecan. Chemotherapy uses chemicals to kill cancer cells, but in the process, it may also damage normal, healthy cells, putting her at an increased risk for developing secondary cancers later in life. It is not guaranteed that the tumor will respond to the chemotherapy that is being used. The treatment plan must constantly be changed, as tumors develop a resistance to specific types of chemotherapy over time.

Chemotherapy often causes mouth sores, pains within the mouth, or excess spit. These conditions can be eased by swishing magic mouthwash (made with Maalox/Mylanta, Benadryl, and Lidocaine), which should be made by the pharmacy, or Orajel mixed with mouthwash. Mouth sores can be treated with an herbal extract called Golden Seal.

Paris contracted thrush and mucositis, which is a contagious disease; caused by fungus (candida albicans) and typically occur in individuals who have a weakened or suppressed immune system due to chemotherapy. The small white eruptions on the mouth, throat, and/or tongue can be treated with Nystatin or fluconazole. To ensure the condition doesn't return patients need to swish four times a day for the full 14 days.

***

Those dreaded words, "I'm sorry, your daughter has cancer." Never in a million years would I think that I would be that parent. Sometimes things can change drastically within seconds. The world is actually a dangerous place where bad things can happen, things that you never dreamed of. From a father's perspective after having a daughter for the first time, the thought typically is, "This is my daughter, and I'm going to dedicate my life to protecting her and saving her from anything harmful." When Ralph learned of Paris' diagnosis, he lost that ability to protect her from anything because he simply didn't have control over this.

One of the memorable things that one of my "cancer mom" friends said to me early on, as she happened to be a veteran in this, is, "It will get easier, you will learn things along the way, and sooner or later you will be telling them what to do." That advice, even though it didn't seem like it at the time, came to be true. I have become my daughter's advocate. I have become knowledgeable about medical decisions in ways that I never thought I would be, and over time, it has gotten easier, as it has become part of my life. One of the main things that I want to stress is that Paris is first and foremost an individual. She has cancer, but cancer doesn't control her, nor should it control any other child. Cancer doesn't primarily control our family lives either. It's an unfortunate part of our lives, but it doesn't lessen our level of hope or dictate how we live, how we spend our finances, and the goals we strive for. We as people adapt to change – we may not like situations that arise, but we have no other choice but to deal with what we encounter.

When we were given an option, we had to choose from two evils: do we want to try and fight this or plan for her funeral? To us, quality of life was a very important factor when considering treatment options. I personally had to put myself in Paris' place and say to myself, if I had cancer and my mother had to decide what was best for me, would I be grateful that I was alive but with limitations? I said that we will fight to the very end, but I wouldn't be selfish either, considering the quality of life every step of the way. I want her to have a quality of life and not be resentful that she can't have a "normal life." I have had to prioritize certain things that I'd be willing to sacrifice, such as her hearing, vision, cognitive functioning, energy level, height, mobility issues, endocrine issues, ability to reproduce, or the necessity of certain organ function. I find myself asking Ralph what are we going to do, and his response is always, "What we have to do." Life is going to do what it's going to do. I learned that you can't plan.

Chapter 6: Effects of Chemotherapy

Everyone says there is no manual for raising children. Many unexpected situations occur that you have no idea how to deal with. There is definitely not a manual out there for raising a child with cancer. You make the best decisions, and most of the time it is trial and error. It is an extremely difficult situation. You make decisions based on your current knowledge, research, and gut-wrenching feeling you have at the time and hope and pray for the best outcome.

Over the course of Paris' treatment, we had to make many of those difficult decisions. One of those came when we decided to enroll Paris in a treatment study. Before she began, we had to sign an "experimental subject agreement." Through the study, the team would take tumor samples and document Paris' case as she participated in the treatment plan. Anytime you enter a study, you need to ask yourself, will entering this study jeopardize my chances of entering future studies? If so, how long will I need to wait to enroll in another study?

Debating on when to start treatment is a scary thing when surgeries get put on hold, treatment becomes delayed due to low counts, or the treatment plan changes all together. Cancer can't fight itself, and timing is crucial. You think we have to act now; we can't just let it sit there and do nothing. You need to remember, though, that rushing things may not be the best decision. Cancer is complicated, and you need to think strategically to tackle it. Be patient, though, because time does always work things out, even though you may not feel that way at the given moment.

Cancer is unpredictable, because despite the fact that your child looks physically well on the outside, he or she can be suffering internally and still be non-symptomatic. Cancer can change things in an instant.

Whatever treatment decision you make, is it really you making the decision, or is it supposed to lead you back to where you're really designed to be anyway? You can't second guess the decision you make at the time, even if it comes back in a negative manner. You made the decision based on the knowledge you had and the feelings you felt. The decisions you make are actually running the course of the overall plan.

Paris' pathology of her tumor sample was consistent with poorly differentiated neuroblastoma, N-MYC non-amplified, one copy, a ploidy of 1.36 and a favorable histology. DNA ploidy refers to the amount of DNA found in each cell. Cells with the same amount of DNA as normal cells are referred to as diploid. Neuroblastoma cells with increased DNA are called hyperdiploid. Paris was diagnosed with stage 3 paraspinal mass neuroblastoma. Her treatment team decided to first provide Paris with a standard chemotherapy regiment.

Over the course of her chemotherapy, I watched Paris become very sick, vomiting countless times per day despite the use of zofran. I witnessed Paris have countless blood transfusions. I learned how to independently change Paris' dressing, which is the covering for her central line, and flush and clean the line. I watched as her little body withered away into nothing but skin and bones, her color changed into a permanent jaundice yellow, and her eyes sulked with sadness at the constant infusions and tests.

When a patient undergoes chemotherapy, doctors routinely order lab/blood draws called complete blood counts (CBC) to check the patient's counts and determine how the patient is responding to treatment. In Paris' case, this happened at every appointment. It helps the doctors to focus on the cells that circulate within the body. Three of the main cells that are examined are red blood cells, white blood cells (WBC), and platelets. Platelets are formed by bone marrow and are necessary to stop bleeding through the process of clotting. Hemoglobin, (HGB), a protein that carries oxygen in red blood cells, is also closely examined.

Chemotherapy can lead to low red blood cell, white blood cell, and platelet counts. It also decreases the bone marrow's ability to produce new red cells, resulting in low energy, fatigue, and anemia. This also increases the patient's risk for access bleeding. If a patient's hemoglobin falls below 8.0, he or she might need a blood transfusion. Having a platelet count of less than 50 also requires a transfusion.

The absolute neutrophil count (ANC) is the body's ability to fight off infection. Chemotherapy destroys both healthy and diseased cells, making it difficult for the body to fight off infection. Neutropenia means the body has a low amount of neutrophils. The severity of neutropenia depends on the ANC. Mild neutropenia exists when the ANC falls between 1,000 and 1,500, moderate neutropenia is between 500 and 1,000, and severe neutropenia exists when the ANC falls below 500. Children who are neutropenic must remain in isolation, and the individuals around them need to thoroughly wash their hands. Caregivers must monitor their temperatures regularly via mouth, ear, or underarm. Temperatures of children undergoing chemotherapy should never be taken rectally due to bleeding and infection.

Paris needed her first blood cell transfusion on January 31, 2008. The nurse brought up the small unit of blood, the equivalent of a pint. It was very strange to see that they were pumping a stranger's blood into my child. It is said that a newborn's body only has 1 cup of blood, and here Paris, who was only 2 months old, was receiving blood from a donor. Blood transfusions became a regular occurrence after that, and I got used to seeing them bring a bag of blood to our room and hang it from the hook and watching it drip for four hours.

Thank God for blood donors! It's that simple. There are four types of blood: A, B, AB (universal), and O negative (also universal). Every three seconds, someone needs blood. Without people taking 45 minutes to donate blood, there wouldn't be a supply for the 4.5 million individuals who need it to survive. Approximately 32,000 pints of blood are used per year. In order to donate, people must be in good health, 16 years or older and at least 110 pounds. Although 60 percent of the U.S. population is eligible to donate, only 5 percent do on an annual basis.

On December 10, 2007, Paris' hair began to thin, and by February 1, 2008, she was completely bald. It greatly saddened me to watch this process. First it became thinner, where at every touch or stroke; thin layers would instantaneously come out in your hand. I would have chunks of hair just sitting in my hand. As she woke up from naps or as I lifted her from the car seat, remains of her hair would be left behind. Eventually it all fell out evenly and she was completely bald. Her scalp became extremely dry, and I oiled it to remove any dirt that formed. It's amazing when you look into the face of child who is bald – you can solely focus on their eyes and their expressions. Due to different treatment plans, Paris has lost her hair three times, and each time it has come back differently. Paris was born with straight jet black hair, and when it fell out the first time, it came back a bit lighter and curlier. When it fell out the second time, it came back lighter yet, a golden/brown. At first, it grew in straighter from the roots, but then ringlet curls came in underneath. Sometimes I think about how it has taken us so long just to grow her hair back, and in the event of a relapse, it could be gone in an instant.

Paris completed her first chemotherapy regiment on February 1, 2008. From February 11 to 14, Paris underwent MRI, CT, MIBG, and bone scans. The team at Children's Memorial Hospital gave Paris fentanyl, a sedative given to keep younger patients asleep through the imagining. The scans indicated that the tumor had responded to the chemotherapy and shrunk to an operative size, causing its tentacles to retract away from the spinal cord. We attributed this news to the blessings of the Virgin Mary, as she appeared on February 11, 1858, to Bernadette Soubirous at the Grotto of Massabielle in Lourdes, France, Our family saw this as a sign of miracles to come.

Chapter 7: Paris' First Surgery

February was hectic. Many at-home nurses came to our home to drop off supplies and teach me how to care for Paris, dispense all of her medications, give her injections, draw her blood, and monitor her health at home. I created a chart of exactly what materials and syringes I needed in the correct order to deal with her central line. First, I needed to collect all the materials, get a trash can, get alcohol pads and lay out the pump to administer the Neupogen for 30 minutes. I needed the saline, dextrose (D5), Neupogen (G-CSF), saline, and heparin. I needed to remember to tap out all the bubbles from the syringes, flush out the line before and after the Neupogen, and clamp the line after pushing through the substances. Paris could still receive the Neupogen through her broviac, or central line.

With the revolving door of health care professionals came a variety of experience levels. One nurse brought a device to dispense Neupogen at a slow rate, but it seemed as if she was unfamiliar with the pump. She told me that we could learn how to use it together.

Immediately I said, "I don't really feel comfortable with you testing the product's functions on Paris. I need someone out here that knows this pump, so if you don't, just be honest and send someone who does." Another time, a different nurse was sent to draw blood and dropped the vial all over my floor. Finally I got a consistent nurse, Joanna, who was knowledgeable and reliable.

On February 20, 2008, Paris had and passed echo- and audiograms. These are recommended for children who have undergone chemotherapy both before and after the treatment as a baseline to monitor future side effects. An audiogram is a hearing test that measures and records how a person can hear different sounds and frequencies. Children who have undergone specific chemotherapy, such as cisplatin, are at risk for high-frequency hearing loss. An echogram determines the strength of the heart. The test detects sound waves given off by the heart. Children who have undergone a specific chemotherapy, such as doxorubicin, have an increased risk for future heart problems.

Paris underwent surgery on March 6, 2008, with Dr. Marleta Reynolds to remove the tumor in the thoracic area. We stayed at the hospital until March 13, 2008. At only 4 months old, she was given at least six doses of morphine each day to control the pain of just having surgery.

As an inpatient at the hospital, I felt trapped, isolated, scared, and alone. It's sad when the hospital becomes your home. I would have loved to talk to someone other than the nurse that comes in every 30 minutes. We would start a conversation but then have to wait 30 minutes while she made her rounds before we finished the conversation. I didn't shower for three days. I just let myself go because I was so consumed with the events around me. My friend came in to braid my hair so it wouldn't look so oily and dirty. One has to understand that if your child is in the hospital for an extended time, you don't leave her side and your needs become secondary to ensure that you are there for her. The nurses offered to watch Paris so I could get something to eat or get some fresh air, but they also had a floor full of other patients to attend to. At the same time, having visitors can be a blessing as well as an annoyance. It can be tiring to constantly have people in and out and discuss, "How things are going?" when you are mentally, physically, and emotionally exhausted yourself. Having people in and out of the room also unnecessarily exposes your child to germs when they are already in a compromised state, so sometimes it is better just to be isolated to avoid risk.

The hospital was all Paris had ever known. She was born into a hospital, and then nine days later was admitted into another. It was so difficult to watch nurses and doctors enter the room every hour as my baby slept, disrupting her sleep. It became her routine that she would wake up in a panic and then fall back asleep. She couldn't rest comfortably. She was forced to be on the defense.

Just one day after we were discharged, on March 14, 2008, we were admitted into the emergency room. Paris could not breathe and was gasping for air. She was diagnosed with pleural effusion, which meant that her right lung collapsed, and a chest tube was placed to drain the fluid. We were inpatient again for 10 more days. The team put Paris on a total parenteral nutrition (TPN) supplement containing essential nutrients for one month. It arrived in the mail, and I had to mix it with lipids (fats). These were delivered through her Medi-port to infuse her with a liquid diet in attempts to gain weight.

Specific clothing should be designed for infants and children who have broviacs, Medi-ports, or central lines. It was so difficult to remove Paris' entire onesie with the snaps at the bottom or her shirt to get access to the upper right or left chest area to access the line. It would be wonderful to have stylishly designed onesies or shirts with flaps on the upper right or left side that just opened and closed to access the line, maybe a tee shirt with a flap on the outside that can be buttoned for easy access, maybe a loophole sewn into the shirt to keep the tubes from hanging down. It was so difficult to try to hold her down as she squirmed while I first tried to undress her or remove her arm from a specific sleeve. It would save a lot of frustration for the children rather than to completely undress them since they are already terrified of the initial needle stick.

When a child has a central line, the catheter branches out into tubes or lumens that hang on the outside of the body so that chemotherapy drugs and transfusions can be infused. One time, the tubes got stuck on the zipper of my shirt, and I asked aloud, "What is that?"

Paris answered, "It's my tubies," referring to the tubes that hang from the central line. Then Paris looked at me and said, "It's not easy," and shook her head. It broke my heart. As a mother listening to your child say these types of things, it is so difficult because there is nothing you can say to make it better.

I know of one mother who sewed a pocket on the inside of her child's shirt to hold the tubes so that they wouldn't hang. Another mother had the child wear a sports bra and put the tubes under the elastic. For Paris and other infants, there has got to be a better way than struggling with clothing that is not appropriate for the medical situation. I know Paris liked to tug on the tubes, as she probably thought they were some kind of rattle or toy put there for her entertainment. She naturally wanted to see them and tried to pull them out. Outta sight outta mind is the motto with young children and broviacs.

Chapter 8: A Little Freedom and Then We Started All Over Again

After attending my 10-year high school reunion in April 2008, I thought about my high school experience. I went to an all-girls Catholic high school. I could have gone anywhere in Chicago for high school, but I ended up there, which led me to cross paths with a girl named Jessica. We were friends in high school but then drifted apart after I transferred out my senior year. I bumped into her at the reunion, and we began talking about our lives – what we had done and where we had ended up. We started talking about our families and if we had children. I started saying that I had a daughter who was undergoing treatment for neuroblastoma, not at all expecting her to know what I was talking about. She looked at me and said she knew exactly what that was because her daughter was also diagnosed, at 2 weeks old. Needless to say, this rekindled our friendship and I mentally placed her on my "cancer mom" list. I reflected on the fact that I was supposed to meet her again at that specific point in my life. We didn't have to attend the reunion, but for some reason, we were both there. She had a purpose to be there that night, and in my eyes, it was solely for me to share a story of hope.

Paris had her first post-treatment scan on June 25, 2008. I remember going into Children's Memorial and immediately seeing new faces. They all had their three-ringed "induction" binders, which symbolizes that you are new to the cancer journey. I thought about how that was once me. I walked around with that binder as if it were gold, relying on it for everything. Now I have everything memorized, and I no longer need the binder.

The preliminary scans indicated no evidence of disease, and Paris' team decided that on July 16 her central line could be removed. She would have no broviac, and our overall plan was to just enjoy life with the thought that we could finally put this horrific event behind us. The nurse manager also contacted me in June to say she'd be closing out Paris' file after the clean set of scans. I remember feeling so relieved to think this would be behind us.

I spent the month of August consulting with an orthopedic team about interventions to correct the curvature in Paris' spine. She underwent x-rays and was fitted for a Thoraco-Lumbar Sacral Orthosis (TLSO) brace since the tumor's impact had compromised her spine.

In September, Paris had her first ear infection. I was so happy to have put the cancer behind us and experience this normalcy. Quickly, though, I would realize how naïve I was to think this.

***

Paris was scheduled to have her second post-surgery MRI scan of the spine on September 27, 2008. The team examined the image of the spine and happened to catch a glimpse of a suspicious enhancement in the cerebellum, throwing everyone off guard. Compared to the population of children that they serviced, it was highly uncommon for a patient to relapse in the brain. About 15 minutes after Paris and I left the hospital, I received a phone call from Dr. Morrison. She was quiet at first and then said, "Lauren I have something to tell you. The spine looks good, but there is a new spot in her brain." I pulled into the parking lot of Tony's Grocery on Elston – a landmark that will be engraved in my mind forever.

On October 3, 2008, Paris had an MRI of the brain, which confirmed a 3 centimeter mass in the cerebellum. The cerebellum controls movement and coordination. Tumors in the cerebellum may impair walking, fine motor activities involving leg and arm movements, and speech. Recurrent neuroblastoma brings fewer medical treatment options than the initial diagnosis. The doctors had to devise a plan and consult with their team to decide on the next steps of treatment. I realized quickly that we would be back to dealing with the aspects of cancer and Paris' file would have to be opened again. The call to our nurse case manager to let her know that Paris had relapsed was one of the hardest calls I ever had to make. When she answered, she quickly asked how Paris was. I wanted to say she was doing great, but instead I had to inform her of the bad news.

In its description of neuroblastoma, the American Cancer Society says it "rarely develops in the brain or spinal cord." Well, Paris' neuroblastoma had spinal cord compression, which meant that the tumor had grown and pressed on the spinal cord, and it relapsed in the cerebellum. The cells that were in the spinal fluid could then travel past the blood brain barrier into any area of the brain, and they happened to settle in the cerebellum.

I was terribly upset when I learned of Paris' relapse but needed to remember that we had been down that road before. It taught me that I ultimately needed to begin viewing uneventful periods as simply just being on a break.

When you are dealing with neuroblastoma, you can't get too comfortable. Your family just needs to re-adjust again, as the cancer is really never ending. You need to have courage to face the next day. Our friends James and Carrie once said, "Neuroblastoma erodes our confidence and our hope, but pearls are formed under great adversity. That piece of sand is irritated and irritated, but it ultimately creates something very rare, precious, and hopeful." Do not get stuck in grief. Give yourself time to grieve, and set a time limit. Then, after you have given yourself the chance to be upset, get mad and get ready to fight. The stress that cancer puts on a family is immeasurable, but you need to focus on the positive until they tell you there is nothing else that they can do. Even if you hear that, keep searching. There are always options. Sometimes they are not the options that you like, but there are new developments every day. It is our job to keep our kids alive long enough to receive the treatments.

In my opinion, one of the hardest things to do is waiting for someone to advise you on your next steps when you as a parent know that there are harmful cancer cells lurking within your child. The initial reaction is to do something immediately as every minute counts. However, I also understood the importance of approaching this type of disease with a strategic plan.

On October 8, 2008, we consulted with a renowned, highly respected neurosurgeon from Children's Memorial. The team proposed that we continue with chemotherapy in hopes that the tumor will respond, as they had exhausted all of the options available to her locally. The team in Chicago offered to conduct cranial/spinal radiation to rid any remaining tumor, however the trade off would be unbearable to us. At only 9 months old, the radiation would leave Paris severely cognitively impaired and with limited mobility. With this proposed treatment plan, we would have Paris in body, but not in spirit, which sparks the infamous quality of life that cancer parents are forced to have. She relapsed in the central nervous system (CNS), and our home hospital was wonderful but just not equipped nor experienced with treating this form of the disease. Collaboration was the key for us.

Ralph and I felt we needed to seek out a second opinion. I highly recommend doing this. Don't be afraid to tell the doctors that you disagree with something and want to question their rationale or motive for what they are recommending. You are your child's best advocate and know your child's limits, and you can feel when something's not right.

The truth is that all great minds do not work under the same roof, and if they did, we would be one step closer to finding a cure. Great minds are spread out throughout different facilities. What one specialist believes is the best approach, another may not. It's your obligation as a parent to search out the opinions of others to make the most educated decisions regarding your child's care. The process involves asking another cancer specialist or facility to review the patient's medical records and history. It's important to confirm pathology results and stage of cancer and discuss the best approach in terms of challenges and alternatives to the plan.

Second opinions are especially valuable when one resides in a small rural area where oncology specialists may not be readily available or the type of disease is not commonly present and may need highly specialized or complicated care. They are also valuable even if they just confirm what you already know. I am a strong believer of second opinions, and in my gut, I didn't believe that Paris would make it through another four months of standard chemotherapy. I began to call every cancer treatment center I could find, trying to locate a facility with experience in treating central nervous system (CNS) neuroblastoma, hopefully cases similar to Paris', with new innovative technology and treatments, and with a reputable staff.

My task also included researching facilities that offered treatments outside of the standard measure of care, which is the drug or treatment considered to be the most accepted, widely used, and most appropriate by experts for a particular type of cancer. These facilities focused on experimental/clinical/investigational type of treatment plans.

Clinical trials involve investigational measures not approved by the Food and Drug Administration (FDA) for universal standard care. Participating does not inhibit your child from receiving medical care if you should decide to withdraw from the study at any time. Trials have specific guidelines, such as patient's age, stage of cancer, and previous treatment plans. They are controlled research study groups involving patients and divided into four phases:

- Phase 1 trial drugs have been tested in the lab or on mice but the side effects on patients are not yet known. This is generally not a smart place to start, because they are considered more of an investigative route. Doctors want to gather a small population and provide a low dose to determine the effect. The main purpose is the "take off" stage to test the safety of the drug in the human population, test toxicity, and gather information and data to determine if there is a therapeutic benefit and if a Phase 2 is possible.

- Phase 2 clinical trials investigate whether or not the drug works. The group has a larger population of patients with cancers that have not responded to standard care or treatment protocols.

- Phase 3 trials often include a very large population, and the groups are randomized. There are two groups within Phase 3: controlled and uncontrolled. Controlled groups receive the standard/accepted treatment and uncontrolled groups get the treatment that is under study. Your child could be placed in either group. The FDA usually won't approve a study that hasn't gone through Phase 3.

- The final phase is when the drug or therapy being studied is considered investigational before the FDA has decided that is can be considered safe and effective to be marketed in the United States for a specific use.

Tomorrow's standard measure of care will greatly result from the patients participating in today's clinical trials. The FDA may approve a certain drug as standard measure of care for one type of treatment, however deem it investigational when in combination with other drugs.

Children Memorial Hospital was very helpful in offering resources and directing us to hospitals that offered alternative forms of experimental treatment. We were very fortunate to have a pleasant experience with Children's Memorial Hospital in Chicago. The staff was very open and honest about the treatments they had to offer Paris at the time as well as to discussing alternative protocols they felt would benefit her if we should choose to seek out another facility. I truly felt that they cared about Paris enough to allow us to try whatever necessary rather than keeping her under their care knowing there may be something more beneficial to her elsewhere. It's important for hospitals to know their limitations and work in collaboration with other facilities. I have heard testimonies from other families that their home hospitals were reluctant to allow their patients to travel to other facilities and receive treatment. Some families I have met felt that once they made the decision to seek a second opinion and try another method of treatment, they were abandoned by their home hospital.

When choosing a treatment facility, you need to feel comfortable with the plan of attack and feel supported. You need to be in a place where honesty exists, where doctors will not give you false hope. Our doctors at Children's Memorial said, "What she needs, we can't offer. You need to seek out another facility. What we can offer will just prolong her life and will affect her quality of life." It is very important for facilities to recognize what they can and can't offer. I greatly respect the honesty that was provided to me, as time is very valuable. That honesty allowed me to seek out Memorial Sloan-Kettering and provide Paris with the care she needed.

With the ongoing communication from the oncology team at Children's, I decided that Memorial Sloan-Kettering Center in New York City was the best facility to meet Paris' needs; however, there was one stipulation. They wanted Paris' tumor to be removed before she could participate in their clinical and investigation treatment plans. This posed a conflict because the respected neurosurgeon at Children's wanted to conduct more chemotherapy.

I was running out of time and needed to make a decision, but at that point my hands were tied. Total body radiation was not an option. I couldn't fly Paris to New York to have the surgery done at Memorial Sloan-Kettering because she wasn't a candidate to fly with a 3 centimeter tumor. I was at a loss. Then, out of the blue, we found a neurosurgeon named Tord Alden who was willing to remove the tumor. This man saved Paris' life – period. He took on a challenge that the "best" wouldn't. He gave her the opportunity to travel to New York to try alternative treatments. I believe that Paris would have died if she had gone through another four months of chemotherapy.

Approximately 30,000 to 40,000 children are undergoing treatment for childhood cancer in the United States. It is the leading cause of death by disease in children under the age of 15 in the United States. In fact, every 16 hours a child with neuroblastoma dies, yet there is a lack of funding and awareness by society and pharmaceutical companies in relation to pediatric cancer, specifically neuroblastoma.

My friend Fran said, "By only sticking with what drugs are going to sell the most or make the most profit, we are robbing our littlest victims a fair fight." The FDA has only approved two new drugs for pediatric cancer use in the past 20 years: Tenoposide (Vumar/VM-26-BMS) in 1990 and Clofarabine (Clolar-Genzyme) in 2004 for acute lymphocytic leukemia (ALL) (www.maxsringoffire.org). July 9, 2012, became a historical moment for children suffering from pediatric cancers as the Creating Hope Act, Section 908 of the FDA Safety and Innovation Act of 2012, was signed into law by President Obama as the first legislation to address the need for new drugs to be developed for children with cancer and other life-threatening diseases.

Chapter 9: Lack of Funding

Lack of money and funding limits finding a cure, and time is running out for children affected by neuroblastoma. Hope lies with private institutions, generous donors, and dedicated researchers who have made it their goal to discover more effective treatments and hopefully find a cure. Their mission is to help the children affected today and those who will be unfairly chosen to fight tomorrow. Neuroblastoma is the most common cancer in infants but receives less than 1 percent of federal funding. The National Cancer Institute budget in 2003 was $4.6 billion. Of that, breast cancer received 12 percent of funding, prostate 7 percent and all 12 major groups of pediatric cancer received less than 3 percent.

Numerous organizations focus on cancer research and make many fundraising attempts, but it is important to know when getting involved with certain groups exactly where and how the donations will be distributed. In 2009, the American Cancer Society provided $0.007 (less than a penny) to childhood cancer research for every dollar of public support, yet it is an "official sponsor of birthdays." How many birthdays are we going to celebrate if only 0.6 percent of fundraising is allotted to pediatric cancer research? Many families support Relay for Life as a method to raise funds for childhood cancer research. However, when you examine the numbers closely, the fundraising efforts are not distributed in the methods in which you may have thought. In 2010 the American Cancer Society posted a pie graph labeling where its fundraising efforts go: 72 percent are used for program services, including 28 percent for patient support, 16 percent for research, 16 percent for prevention and 12 percent for detection/treatment. The remaining 28 percent of the fundraising efforts includes 21 percent for fundraising efforts and 7 percent for management and general administration. If one should participate in Relay for Life and raise $1,000, 28 percent ($280) will go toward administration and fundraising costs. Only $160 (16 percent) will go toward any research, and $6 (0.6 percent) of that $1,000 raised will go toward childhood cancer. Commonly one will hear the debate that research into adult cancers can benefit children, however, many adult cancers do not affect our children. They have their own types of specific childhood cancers that need specific fundraising efforts.

The National Cancer Institute (NCI), formed under the National Cancer Institute Act of 1937, is the federal government's principal agency for cancer research and training. Why is the federal funding amount for prostate cancer, with a 99 percent five-year survival rate, nearly five times the total given to all types of childhood cancer? A fellow cancer parent once told me, "Think of cancer as a sinking ship with all of us on board. Who do we care for first? It's said to get the women and children out first to safety. We know that any mom would give up her seat for her child. Why then are we giving first-class seating (funding) to adults?"

Some organizations that contribute specifically to childhood cancer–related causes or research for neuroblastoma are parent-based organizations such as Cookies for Cancer in combination with GLAD, Alex's Lemonade Stand, Arms Wide Open, Cure Search, The Rally Foundation for Childhood Cancer Research, Mystic Foundation, and the Band of Parents organization, which supports the world's largest cancer treatment centers with funds to conduct treatments and research in hopes to find the long awaited cure for neuroblastoma.

Many of these foundations were created by parents with the overall consensus that it is unacceptable for kids to get cancer. We as parents have common goals...to advocate so that things can be done better and increase awareness for funding so treatments that are already there waiting to be produced can be financially supported. Dr. Cheung from Memorial Sloan-Kettering told me that a humanized antibody that could improve treatments would cost between $1 million and $2 million to fund.

The Truth 365 is an Emmy-award winning documentary film and social media campaign that "gives a voice to kids fighting cancer."

The collaborative campaign is led by Arms Wide Open Childhood Cancer Foundation, Melinda Marchiano, Frankie's Mission, Journey 4 A Cure, The Rally Foundation, and Emmy-award-winning producer Mike Gillette. The goal is to educate and mobilize millions of people through social media networking to inform the public of the critical need for funding for pediatric cancer research. Our personal journey is documented in the Truth 365 in attempts to inspire others to join the cause. "Helping children with cancer and other life-threatening illnesses should be a national priority." The Gabriella Miller Kids First Research Act (H.R 2019) would require the director of the National Institutes of Health to allocate $126 million to $12.6 million each year for 10 years of appropriated funds for pediatric research. This bill, honoring Gabriella Miller, was passed by the House on December 11, 2013, in a bipartisan 295-103 vote. This important legislation was also passed by the Senate in March 11, 2014. The bill was signed into law on April 3, 2014 by President Obama.

The Ronald McDonald House collects pop tops to assist with ongoing costs within the facility. We have many people collect for us during the year, and then at the end of the year, we drop them off to designated locations where they are sent to recycling centers and cashed in. The Ronald McDonald House estimates that 1,267 pop tops equals approximately 1 pound, which earns between 50 and 75 cents. I collected approximately 69,685 pop tops (55 pounds) in one year. At 75 cents per pound, that meant I donated $41.25 to the Ronald McDonald House. The Ronald McDonald House estimates that 63,360 pop tops equal one mile in length. It's amazing to think that we donated enough pop tops to exceed 1 mile. It doesn't seem like much, but when numerous people are collecting for a cause, it becomes significant. The largest Ronald McDonald House was located in New York on 73rd street until June 28, 2012, when the Chicago location opened a house containing 14 floors with 86 rooms for families.

The 10th annual MIX radiothon in 2010 raised $1.6 million for Children's Memorial Hospital, and it makes me feel so proud that we were a part of that. We shared our story, and so many people listened. It was touching to hear that people are looking at things in a new perspective and light. Our story motivated people to donate and help children who are battling illnesses every day. My story that was difficult to share touched people's hearts. During the interview, which can be found on YouTube, I stated that Paris is the strongest person I know. She handles this situation better than I do at times. She goes with the flow, as it has unfortunately become a normal part of her life. She really doesn't have many complaints.

We have been blessed by the many efforts done specifically for Paris since her diagnosis. Many friends, families, strangers, and co-workers have come together to brainstorm fundraising efforts to aide in the ongoing medical costs that she will endure over her lifetime. My mother works at Northwestern Memorial Hospital and organized an annual holiday cookie sale in honor of Paris. Everyone in her department participates and bakes dozens of cookies to sell. The sale happens around the Christmas holidays, and staff members bring in cookie containers to fill for the holidays.

There were so many companies that were willing to assist us with fundraising events, and there were countless restaurants, businesses, and spas that were willing to donate a percentage of their sales earned on a given fundraising day to our cause. I have meet people who make jewelry who offered to have jewelry parties and have had handcrafted cards made and sold in honor of Paris. People have hosted Avon, Tastefully Simple, Origami Owl, Thirty-One Bags, and Pampered Chef parties for Paris. People have held bake sales, held raffles with donated prizes for auction items, raffled off their time shares for a week's stay, donated a new Wii and other prizes. We held fun fairs, golf events, and bags tournaments. We sold rubber bracelets to honor Paris, made T-shirts to sell and made lanyard pins with the cancer ribbon engraved with Paris' name and birthdate. We sold cookbooks containing a variety of recipes from all of our friends. One author did a book signing and donated the proceeds to Paris. Both local and out of state bands – Echo-Field, Zero, When All Else Fails, and The Killers – held shows in honor of Paris and donated the proceeds. Our Lady of Mercy Church in Aurora and countless other churches have Paris on their prayer lists.

Kara, a 5th grade student at Johnson Elementary, was so touched and inspired by Paris' story that she independently organized a St. Baldrick's event for Paris in which Fox News attended. She had been saving for months for an American Girl Doll and finally had $91.14, but instead of buying a doll, she donated all of it to Paris. Joseph Academy schools took it upon themselves to organize Pennies for Paris, where teachers arranged with their principals and collected money from staff on Friday in exchange for wearing jeans that day.

People have also just donated money for no reason at all. I called to request additional coupons through Enfamil, and after sharing Paris' story, the representative could relate on a personal level. Instead of sending me coupons, she sent me an entire case of formula to help us out financially. It's people like these who make a difference in our already stressful lives. Their little acts of kindness have touched my heart and will always be remembered. All of these efforts do take time and work. It required making connections, speaking out, being proactive by writing letters, and sharing her story, but by doing so I got a tremendously generous response. I have created friendships with some of the people that I have dealt with who genuinely care about Paris and her journey.

Chapter 10: The Eagerness to Help

During the first week of October 2008, Paris underwent a number of scans at Children's Memorial, including a CT of the chest, abdomen, and pelvis and an MRI of the brain and spine. The days were very busy and long. Paris was sedated daily. They used all of her veins since she no longer had her central line. They used an IV overnight, but it left her with a severe rash/hives because she is allergic to the tegaderm – adhesive tape they used. Many of the veins in her arms, hands, and feet were blown. This loving and caring mom that I thought that I would be had to turn somewhat cold and tell her to be brave and focus, constantly telling her that she's a good girl and then listening to her repeat it, "I good girl," with tears running down her face, as she has just been stuck by needles. It's the worst feeling in the world knowing you can't save her.

The tests showed that the growth from the residual tissue was most likely neuroblastoma. Her liver hid the tumor, causing the MIBG scan not to light up in that area. It instead lit up in the cerebellum, confirming that the tumor had spread and settled in her cerebellum (3 centimeters). There was a high probability that it was in the central location as well.

At this time the tumor was just resting against the cerebellum, which is why she was still moving, crawling, and standing with no symptoms or complications. If she were to begin exhibiting symptoms such as twitching, jerking, or being unable to move her legs or feet, then they would implement a shunt to relieve the pressure caused by the tumor.

An MRI of the brain and a CT scan helped the doctors see if any other parts were affected. The final test was the bone marrow, where they needed to remove a portion of Paris' hip bone from the right and left side to determine if the cancer had spread to her bones. A bone marrow aspiration is where small pieces of the bone, marrow, and fluid are taken from the front and back of the pelvic bone. Memorial Sloan-Kettering takes bone marrow aspirations from four sites – two from the front and two from the back – to gather a more extensive sample. It takes three to four days to test and dissect the bone.

The doctors told us that the percentage of kids with neuroblastoma is small, the percentage of kids who have tumors that return is even smaller, and the percentage of kids who have them return in such an aggressive manner as Paris' is nearly next to none.
Their plans included clinical trials, chemotherapy combinations, and treatment regiments that were still being tested to treat recurrent cancer. Basically we were making up the treatment plans as we went and hoped that it worked. Also, since she already had chemo to treat her 7 centimeter tumor, her body likely wouldn't respond positively to it this time, so we needed to find another course of treatment.

After researching on my own and calling the top cancer research hospitals in the country (MD Anderson, St. Jude, Mayo Clinic, Golisano Children's Hospital, City of Hope, Dana-Farber, and UIC Cancer Center), we determined (without knowing all of the test results) that the best treatment option for us may be in New York at Memorial Sloan-Kettering. It has four pediatric oncologists specializing in neuroblastoma and has used clinical trials, including an at-the-time new development using iodine 131 and antibodies 3F8. The antibodies find tumor cells and carry tumor-killing substances to the neuroblastoma without harming the normal cells. I wasn't sure how it would work with the blood brain barrier, but according to the literature, Paris was a candidate. The blood brain barrier is a barrier between the blood and the tissue of the central nervous system that keeps toxins from entering the brain. A type of chemotherapy known as Temodar can cross the blood brain barrier.

After hearing this bit of hope from Sloan-Kettering, we thought that was just what we needed. We were willing to travel wherever necessary to get Paris the best treatment possible. All I knew was that she was strong, and now we had these possibilities.

Chapter 11: Welcome to New York

Paris underwent her first brain surgery on October 13, 2008. The surgeon successfully removed ALL of the visible tumor without damaging a significant part of the cerebellum. The entire surgery lasted more than five hours. Under the circumstances, this was the best news that we could have heard. She would need to undergo physical therapy later in life to re-strengthen her left side, focusing on coordination. But that day, she conquered the first of many steps and was doing fine. I was able to see her fresh incision which was approximately 10 inches in length. My daughter's brain was just tampered with and now held together by hundreds of stitches and staples. She would need an MRI scan to confirm that the tumor was removed. The plan was to then do two more surgeries – one to insert an Ommaya reservoir in her brain for the antibody treatment and one to insert a port in her chest for chemotherapy treatments.

Sloan-Kettering has a world-renowned multidisciplinary team dedicated to treatment and finding a cure. We flew to New York to meet with Dr. Kramer on Tuesday, October 21, 2008, to discuss focal radiation. We decided to cancel the surgeries to place the Ommaya reservoir and port until we heard all of our options.

The day I became a mother the word sacrifice had a new meaning. I can't believe that this is happening and that I'm going through this sometimes. I am doing everything possible and in my power to provide her with the best medical care there is to offer to provide her with the best chance of survival.

I vividly remember our first trip to Sloan-Kettering in New York City. We were at the airport, and our luggage was well over the weight limit. We obviously had over-packed because we didn't know how long we would have to stay or what we would need. Our bags weighed more than 50 pounds, which would have cost $150 per bag. But little acts of kindness go a long way. The gentleman at the airport chose not to charge us for our heavy bags to save us a little cash. He did something so small, but I can't tell you how memorable that act was. I have noticed that since we have endured this situation, people have shown us kindness and humanity on countless occasions.

Over the next few days, we would become familiar with the hospital that would be our resource in attempting to save Paris. The ninth floor, where all the pediatric cancer patients were being treated, is an environment I will never forget. The floor was filled with parents and their children; displaying so many emotions. Many children who were thin and hairless, some weak and some filled with energy despite it all. Almost every child in the ward was attached to an IV pole linked with a bag containing a blood transfusion, platelets, or chemotherapy.

We flew back to Chicago on Wednesday, October 22, after our consultation with Dr. Kramer. We met with everyone on the team over a four-hour period. After long discussions and an evaluation of Paris, they decided that the best treatment option for her long-term health and independent living would be to do focal radiation to the specific area at a low dose of 20 grey over a four-week period beginning that Monday. They felt this would leave little side effects that would only be detected by a neurological test, not by people in her everyday life.

The team had never performed focal radiation on an infant with neuroblastoma, but with their expertise, they felt they could give her low doses of focal radiation and increase the amount of antibody therapy to compensate for the typical protocol of cranial/spinal radiation. Paris would be sedated daily and given 10 minutes of direct radiation to her cerebellum.

The first week in New York would focus on preparing for the treatment, including getting a head immobilizer, putting in a port for future chemo treatments, and doing routine blood draws to determine Paris' counts and the possible need for transfusions. This protocol was seen as the best and only possibility for her survival. This was the only known course of successful treatment. If we did not agree to it, multiple lesions could form on Paris' brain, and they would ultimately be inoperable.

Dr. Kramer informed me that of the approximately 650 documented cases of neuroblastoma in the United States each year, two-thirds are toddlers and older with advanced stage 4 cancer, and only 50 out of the 650 are born with or diagnosed with neuroblastoma before the age of 1. However, Paris' case is considered rare to be born with neuroblastoma with negative MYNC (meaning not high risk) at a stage 3 cancer that developed into an aggressive cancer in her cerebellum. The doctors are baffled by this because there are limited statistics to compare to. The plan was for Paris to receive chemotherapy in Chicago after radiation had been given in New York. She would then return to New York for antibody treatment.

We flew back to New York on Halloween, and Ralph and I stayed at the Ronald McDonald House. Families receiving medical care can stay at the house at a discounted rate compared to the hotels near the hospital. Memorial Sloan-Kettering is on York and 68th, in the heart of Manhattan, where an average hotel stay runs $200-250 per night. It is filled with 84 families, all battling cancer. We were forced to learn our surroundings very quickly. It was sort of like being dropped off and fending for ourselves in a strange environment. We had to rely on our survival skills and adapt, but I was amazed at how quickly I learned.

The staff at the Ronald McDonald House is wonderful and genuinely care about the kids, families, and siblings who stay there. Paris made a lot of friends over the years, and many of her memories center around being there, since our stays varied in duration. Over time, we started to subconsciously call the Ronald McDonald House "home." I feel very fortunate that there are places designed for families who need a place to stay during times of medical treatment, however it is a difficult concept to adjust to. I was very overwhelmed and fairly new to the cancer world. I witnessed parents who had already become accustomed to their new cancer-revolving lifestyle. At first glance, I felt like I had lost everything that I worked for, questioning how I ended up there. This transition was extremely difficult for me, leaving everything I once had. I had to leave behind the person that I once knew. When the staff showed me our room, I felt like I was going backward, reverting to an apartment-sized space with the mere basics: a bathroom and a bedroom. Under the circumstances, I wish places like this didn't have to exist, but I am fortunate to have these places to go.

The house has a very family-orientated atmosphere. Everyone looks out for each other's best interest, and I really feel a sense of belonging, even if this is not the ideal group to belong to. There is a sense of comfort and normalcy because everyone is battling the same fight. Everyone can relate to one another, and half the time they can finish the phrase that you began. The playroom is always open, and countless people are working on crafts and projects. The kids have such a good time that I wondered if Paris would be bored and expect activities all of the time when we returned home. Kids here have a true understanding and compassion for kids who are sick. They really do nurture them and are not afraid of what is out of the norm.

I used to worry that Paris would go to school and think, what's wrong with all of these kids, what is on top of their heads? She has had such a limited exposure to hair that it almost seemed foreign to her. I also am so used to seeing her defined face that I would wonder, when the hair grows back, would she look like another child?

The house supplies its residents with dinners every night. As someone who stayed there, I truly appreciated this, because I would go to the hospital early in the morning and sometimes stay for 8 or 10 hours a day. Can you imagine having to come back and cook? I was so grateful for that, but it was kind of funny because we were subject to whatever they happened to be serving, which often entailed pasta. Each family had one refrigerator shelf on which they could store their own food, but that greatly limited what we could buy and eat.

The house coordinates many V.I.P activities for children and families. We were blessed to do so much while in New York, but I would give it all up in a heartbeat and opt never to do anything fun and expensive if it meant she were healthy.

We were fortunate to take pictures in Central Park with a professional photographer named Chris while Paris looked very healthy for the first time in her life. He treated us like royalty. I have images of Paris, Ralph, and I that I will cherish forever. I wasn't able to take Paris for her monthly photo shoots as an infant because we were always in the hospital. I have pregnancy pictures, a 6-month picture, and 1-year picture, both of which reflect her being sick. I watched her lay in the hospital bed so often that the majority of her pictures from her scrapbook are of her in a hospital gown, have backgrounds of medical devices, heart and respiratory-level monitors, IV poles, an occasional roommate in the background, commonly a nurse, and the overall ugliness of a hospital room. Her album that is supposed to represent her journey through life doesn't consist of pictures of her over the past few years wearing all of the cute outfits that I received at my baby shower. Most of those I never got to use and are still hanging in the closet with the tags still attached. She never wore those clothes because she was always in the "hospital attire," which was an open-back gown that usually was too big for her little body. The scrapbook album that I made for her consists of pictures that reflect the hospital – a place that she has known since 9 days old.

"One accomplishment leads you to the next obstacle."

The Monday of our first week there, Paris was fitted for her radiation mask. Then, on Wednesday, she had routine tests for pre-admission for surgery. On Friday, Paris was to have surgery to implant her Medi-port, which would take two hours. The port is a small appliance implanted beneath the skin toward the upper chest area. It has a dividing wall or partition (a septum) to allow drugs to be given and blood samples to be taken. We arrived at 6:30 a.m. but were not admitted until 7 p.m. because of an emergency surgery. She had been

NPO – ordered to not have any food or liquid – since the night before and was very upset. It was the worst I had ever seen her!

On the days that Paris was NPO, I would have to check little places – her stroller or swing – for snacks and crumbs from previous days. I also ended up waking up multiple times at night just to make sure that I took away the last bottle that she drank at 10 p.m. so that she didn't sneak a few sips after midnight. It never failed that on NPO days I would hear her stir around in her crib. It is heartbreaking to watch and listen to your child beg for food and then cry herself to sleep because she's hungry but cannot have anything the day before scans since anesthesia and sedation is required. I would lie so still in my bed hoping that she would fall back into a deep sleep. After a few minutes of tossing and turning, she must have known that it was midnight because she would be up right away asking for her milk bottle. She continued by saying, "Make it, mama," "Go make it," with tears rolling down her face as she pleaded with me "Mommy, my tummies so empty," and I did nothing.

While in New York, she also had bone marrow tests to ensure that the cancer was not in her bones. The bone marrow in Chicago came back negative, so we hoped this would be a confirmation of the same results. Paris was to begin radiation and a five-day regimen of chemotherapy.

Paris' first week and a half went very well. She experienced a few side effects from the treatment – fatigue and diarrhea – but nothing too bad. The best news that we got was that the bone marrow tests showed no sign of disease in the bones or marrow, meaning one less step of treatment in the future, and ultimately a better outcome for Paris. Her blood counts were also good, higher than 8.0, meaning she didn't need a blood transfusion.

At 11 months old, she was standing for seconds by herself, saying all types of words, and still so active. Our hope was to go home the week of Thanksgiving and start treatment in Chicago on December 1. That would include an intense week of chemotherapy followed by three weeks of isolation. We would then return to New York for three weeks in January for scans. Those would determine whether we continue with the chemo or move onto the antibody treatment.

The many possible outcomes made it hard to plan. Her treatment plan is contingent upon so many things – fever, infection, effects from chemo, common colds, response to chemo, or the possibility of relapse. Dr. Kramer told us she couldn't plan past the three weeks in January but assured us that Paris looked good and was responding well to treatment. I needed to remember *everyday* to take it one day at a time.

Chapter 12: Isolation

The intensive chemotherapy Paris received in Chicago made her really sick after just the first day. The three doses (Carboplatin, Temodar, and Irinotecan) for five straight days really affected her. A specific oral chemo, Temodar, is a gel cap pill that children can usually swallow, however, because of Paris' age; they have to mix the powder with apple juice, but just enough to fill the syringe to ensure that she gets the correct dose. Well, the first attempt was a disaster. As soon as it hit her mouth, the taste was so potent that she threw everything up within seconds. They tried again a while later, and it stayed down after many dry heaves.

On Tuesday we repeated the same thing, so I decided to have them place a nasogastric intubation (NG) tube so that she wouldn't taste it. The tube goes in through the nose, past the throat and down into the stomach. She struggled for 25 minutes and then pulled it out. We repeated the process again, and she pulled it out at home later that night. We had to put another one in on Wednesday, which she finally left alone and I pulled out on Sunday. I also used it to give her Zofran, an anti-nausea medication that has a horrible taste as well.

That week was just horrible, with Paris throwing up everywhere daily – actually hourly – and very tired and moody. On Sunday, she finally had a burst of energy for the first time and didn't vomit. She seemed to be doing a bit better. I hoped it would continue for the next three weeks. She had lost more weight and was down to about 14 and a half pounds. We again had at-home nurse care twice a week to take blood counts. I accessed her port, though, giving her all of her medications and Neupogen daily. When the nurse called to ask if I had any questions or needed a refresher course, I just laughed.

Unfortunately, I'm a professional, I told her.

We spent Paris' isolation period in the hospital. Paris spiked a fever and became neutropenic, with an ANC of 0.8. If during the CBC the doctor finds the ANC to be lower than 500, the child is considered to be neutropenic and should be in isolation. It took me a while to learn to read the reports and know what all of the numbers mean. Individuals who receive either chemotherapy or radiation or both may be at high risk to develop neutropenia at some point. Typically, individuals are at risk seven days after a treatment cycle. Neutropenia is a low number of neutrophils, which are a type of white blood cells. Neutrophils are important because they help to prevent infection within the body. Therefore, when you have an extremely low number, you are at increased risk of infection. In the isolation room, we had to wear protective yellow gowns and wash our hands continuously. Paris could not receive flowers, as they may carry germs. We also had to limit the number of visitors to avoid the spread of contagious germs.

We somewhat expected for her immune system to be compromised or even wiped out due to the dose and type of chemo that she received. Since there are germs and bacteria all around us, Paris was prone to getting sick, whereas the average person could fight off this everyday exposure. Her blood culture determined that she had bacteria in her blood (septicaemia) which typically could be fought off by kids that have had immunizations and haven't just received chemotherapy. She was given antibiotics, but it was not reducing the fevers.

The infectious disease team determined that the bacteria had infected the port. Since it was a foreign object in her body, the bacteria latched onto the port. Because of this, it needed to be removed via surgery. Typically, this would be a minor surgery; however because of her lack of immune system and low white blood counts, she was more prone to infection and would face a longer recovery time. After the port was removed, two IVs infused four different antibiotics into her system to treat the remaining infection.

Children's Memorial only allows one parent to stay by a patient's bedside, but neither Ralph nor I wanted to leave her side. Since our room was a private, isolated room, we had a private adjoining bathroom. The nurses told Ralph that he could obtain a cot and sleep in the family room where second parent typically stays. But Ralph didn't want to leave Paris, or me, at night, so he found a crib mattress in the hallway and laid it on the bathroom floor. He slept there every night for the entire month to be closer to us in case we needed him during the night. Every morning, he would drive 30 minutes to my mom's house to take a shower before going to work.

By that point, we'd had a total of 10 blood/platelet transfusions, which were needed to help reproduce more blood cells and white blood cells. Paris received platelets about twice a day to boost her immune system. As soon as her body absorbed the platelets, they quickly got used. She was up to 75,000 but then dropped to 34,000. We needed to keep her above 50,000. Her red blood cells stayed above 8 and at times reached 11. The white blood cells were beginning to form, but at a count of 2.0, she was still classified as neutropenic.

Her stomach was swollen and extended, measuring 42 centimeters, which put pressure on her lungs, making it difficult to breath. She needed oxygen to help her breathing. X-rays and ultrasounds revealed typhlitis, which causes irritation in the lining of the large intestine, causing diarrhea and pain. The doctors explained that the harsh chemo affected the lining of the organ, and with time, antibiotics and increased white blood cells would help the swelling go down.

Paris continued to have fevers, and it just seemed as if she was not getting any better. The doctors kept reassuring me that whatever she had couldn't be treated. It would just take a while, depending on how quickly her immune system recovered. We were scheduled to return to New York on January 1, but we'd have to wait and see about Paris' condition.

People ask me all of the time, how do you do it? My response is that I just do. I don't know how I do it sometimes. I don't know how I can remember everything so precisely regarding her medical treatment yet I can't remember yesterday. I just do it because I have to – she's counting on me. I'm her advocate. I'm her mom. I question how people don't do everything possible for their child.

As we sat in isolation in December 2008, we learned from the nursing staff that there was a baby found in the cold, left to die, who was just brought into the emergency room alone, scared, hungry, and cold and with no one to care for him. I try to process that, but it seems so unfair. I was fighting to keep my baby alive on a daily basis, and others who are blessed with healthy children are doing things to inflict harm or death without even giving them a chance at life. Just dumping them, waiting for the elements to take control. Not even giving them a chance, by leaving them somewhere where they will be noticed and taken care of by someone who cares. I did everything right and I have a baby who is ill. Again I wouldn't wish this life on anyone, but it seems very unfair.

Some people view it as an honor to be chosen to be the mother of a sick child because God knows that you will do everything in your power to fight for her chance at survival at any cost. After a long conversation with Ralph, I confided in him that sometimes I don't feel like a real mom. I felt like my motherhood has been taken away from me. I told him that all I wanted to do was to be a mom, and I feel like I have been cheated from that treasured part of my life. I think he was the most sincere that I had ever heard him. He really inspired me with his response.

He said, "Lauren, you are the best mother ever. You are doing more than any mother has done in her lifetime."

Chapter 13: Paris' Relapse and Dr. LaQuaglia

Paris and I arrived in New York on January 1, 2009. That week, she had an MRI scan of the brain and spine and a CT scan of the chest, abdomen, and pelvis. Those results would tell the doctors whether or not she needed surgery in the thoracic area on January 8. If the scans showed enhancement due to post-surgery, chemo, and radiation, then she would be declared "cancer free" at that time and could undergo antibody treatment to target any free-floating cells. However, if the doctors saw enhancement due to the tumor, by comparing her current scans with those from September, she would need surgery. If the area changed based on chemo that would mean there was still a tumor. If the area stayed the same that would mean it was most likely scar tissue.

The team, including the oncologists, surgeon, social workers, radiation oncologists, and pathologists, holds conferences on Tuesdays to provide a collective opinion on the situation and devise the best approach in the event of a recurrence. We waited anxiously to hear, hoping that Paris would be cleared for the antibody treatment.

When I finally heard from the doctors, they began by telling me that they had good news. The MRI scans confirmed that the initial site in the thoracic area was in fact neuroblastoma; however it was initially very small. The chemo in December had further decreased it to almost nothing. At the time of the call, they were still debating whether or not to go through with the surgery on the 8th because the area was so small. The team thinks that maybe the antibody will be enough to rid Paris of the disease rather than putting her through surgery.

Initially, they decided to bypass the surgery to remove the remaining neuroblastoma and move forward with implanting the Ommaya and starting treatment with antibody 8H9, a different antibody than what I had researched. However, the next day the doctors found a 4 centimeter mass (neuroblastoma) surrounding the aorta. They believed this to be the original location of the tumor, not the spinal canal, where the 7 centimeter mass was. With that larger mass removed, they could now see the one around the aorta. I was so confused. One day the doctors thought they may not even need to remove the tumor surgically and go straight to the antibody treatment, now we would be undergoing surgery to remove a larger mass that had been detected.

***

People consult with Dr. LaQuaglia when others have told them that the neuroblastoma is inoperable. Imagine that for a second. Imagine facing a life-threatening illness. You have given up everything and have tried every avenue to save your child's life. Then you come to a crossroads. Scan results say the tumor is in an inoperable spot, and the doctors can't do anything more to fight the cancer. They say it's over.

Dr. LaQuaglia doesn't accept that. He is the surgeon that people from all over the world consult with to obtain that second opinion and to seek hope. He is truly considered to be a miracle worker – there is really no other way to describe it. He genuinely cares about the children with whom he works. He puts no time limit on procedures and always states that it will take as long as it takes to get the job done. He searches the area in question to ensure he has gotten as many of the cancer cells as possible.

Dr. LaQuaglia explained that Paris was about to undergo a very serious, life-threatening surgery. That it was more complicated than the brain surgery because if the aorta was clipped, she could have excessive bleeding, causing fatality. Also, the tumor encompasses some of the blood vessels that supply blood to the spinal canal. If these turned out to be the only supply to the spinal cord, Paris could become paralyzed, but that would not be determined until after surgery. The surgeon seemed hopeful that there may be other sources to the spinal region, but he had seen both horrible outcomes happen.

We prayed for a positive, successful surgery to ensure that the team could remove the entire tumor. In the past, her surgeries have resulted in the best possible outcomes, so we were praying that this time would be the same. After the surgery, Dr. LaQuaglia would biopsy the tumor. If the cells were "active," then they would need to radiate that area, leaving us with just one safe dose of radiation left given Paris' weight and age. If the cells are not active, then the team will begin the antibody treatment.

Paris went into surgery with Dr. LaQuaglia at 9:30 a.m. on January 9, 2009, and everything was complete by 7:30 p.m. I sat and waited for 10 hours and trusted the surgeon with her little life in his hands. Ralph had flown to New York the day before to be with us while Paris stayed in the Intensive Care Unit (ICU) for 10 days. We consulted with the doctor after surgery and then waited until they finished up. They took her by ambulance, literally a 3 minute ride across the street to New York Presbyterian Hospital, to closely monitor Paris. By the time we got settled into our room, it was close to 10 p.m.

It was a very long day, and each minute that passed felt like a lifetime, but thankfully, everything went extremely well. The doctor was able to remove the entire visible tumor and stated that he continued to search around the area. He took biopsies of the liver and placed a central line and a port. Paris only lost 50cc of blood, which was good. After surgery, the doctor told us Paris had jerked her arms and legs like she was having a seizure. The scans, however, did not show any brain activity that would indicate one.

She received extra sedation during the night because she kept trying to wake up. During surgery she was purposely paralyzed to prevent movement, and it would take awhile for her to regain feeling. However, even on that first night, when the nurses checked the movement in her legs and feet, they were already responding to touch. It appeared that once again, our girl had overcome major surgery with the best possible outcome, in part because of all the positive thoughts and prayers from others.

I was not mentally prepared to see the image of her after surgery. The staff told me she would be swollen and look "puffy" in addition to being connected to countless monitors and tubes. In actuality, Paris looked like she has been hit by a Mack truck. It was hard to see her sprawled out on the hospital bed, connected to monitors that constantly beeped, bandaged from the waist down and laying lifeless.

After recovering from surgery, Paris would undergo another dose of radiation. When they took biopsies of the area and examined them, they saw a combination of dead tissue from the chemotherapy and "active" neuroblastoma cells, meaning that the chance of reoccurrence was a possibility.

Chapter 14: Antibody 8H9

Paris was scheduled to have the Ommaya placed on January 20 so she could begin antibody treatment. However, the morning of the surgery, our insurance company cancelled what they had already approved. It was very frustrating because Paris had been NPO all day. Paris could tell that I was frustrated, and it becomes evident when your 2 ½ year old tells you not to worry and that everything is going to be alright. Apparently, the way in which the claim was submitted and the individuals who were to process the certification number did not have all of the information, therefore they had to deny the approval. The wording in claims is also very important. My insurance will not cover experimental/clinical trial treatment (which is what antibody treatment was considered). We needed to prove to them that the surgery was not part of the clinical trial, but simply surgery. According to Dr. Kramer, under the experimental clinical trial, the actual antibody and scans directly associated with the antibody are covered under the trial, so that is all that is considered experimental. However, according to insurance, everything associated with the antibody treatment, such as clinic appointments, doctor visits, medications associated with treatment, blood draws, etc., would not be covered. The hospital suggested that if I wanted to proceed with the surgery for that day and not wait for approval, I could put down a $15,000 deposit that day on my credit card. Needless to say I decided to wait for a response from my insurance company.

The very next day, after numerous telephone calls and reviews, the insurance company approved the surgery. Unfortunately, the one day delay meant we needed to reschedule. It also meant another month in New York.

Dr. LaQuaglia took biopsies of Paris' liver and bone marrow. The results were benign, meaning the cancer had not spread to those areas! The bad news was that the actual tumor site still had active neuroblastoma cells; therefore we did a round of chemo – irenotecan, which also crosses the blood brain barrier – to fight the tumor in her brain and focal radiation to the chest area, where her initial disease site presented. We began radiation on January 28, twice a day for seven days, once in the morning and once in the afternoon, leaving her NPO for the majority of the day. The Ommaya placement was rescheduled for February 6, meaning we would have to make up some radiation time to fit in the surgery.

The original plan was for Paris to receive the 8H9 antibody treatment on February 17 and again February 24. Now we would not begin antibody treatment until March. After the placement of the Ommaya, Paris would receive an entire week of nuclear medicine scans. Dr. Kramer suggested that we extract Paris' stem cells toward the end of the month.

My plan was to return to work in March, but I learned that I would need to be in New York on March 2 for Paris' antibody 8H9 treatment. The stay would be at least another three weeks. The second antibody 8H9 treatment would be March 17, followed by an MRI of the brain and spine as well as team meetings. Further treatment would be determined from there. Besides that, Paris was so sick from treatment and so tired. I was so busy with countless people that I had to remain in contact with for her care. Paris had also gotten rotavirus, a highly contagious virus that causes an infection within the digestive tract, causing her to be fatigued and dehydrated, exhibit chronic vomiting, and have high fevers. Since she never obtained the Prevnar vaccine and had been subject to chemotherapy, she was susceptible to contacting the illness.

She was on so many medications that my room looked like a pharmacy. She was primarily on Pentamidine, Nystatin, Zofran, Megestrol, and Fluconazole, and she would fight me when it was time to take them. As soon as she saw them coming toward her in the syringe, she would tighten her lips, swing her arms and say, "NO!" in a strong assertive tone. It was rough – being alone for such a long time and managing everything by yourself, not ever being able to take a break, being constantly surrounded by situations that physically and emotionally drain you.

On February 6, 2009, Dr. Souweidane, a pediatric neurosurgeon from Weill Cornell Medical College in New York, implanted the Ommaya reservoir on the right side of Paris' frontal lobe. An Ommaya reservoir is an intraventricular catheter system used to deliver chemotherapy into the cerebrospinal fluid. It consists of one lateral ventricle attached to a reservoir implanted under the scalp.

The surgery went great, and Paris was recovering well. She touched her head and noticed a bump and didn't try to touch it again. It looked as if she bumped her head and had a bruise. Her hair would grow over it and cover it. It is permanent. It will never come out. We stayed in the hospital for 24 hours, and Paris had a CT scan to ensure proper placement. We were to go back in 7 to 10 days to get the stitches removed. On February 7, we went in for the CFS (Flow Study), where they inject dye to ensure that the antibody will flow properly. The dye injection kit was supposed to arrive by 1 p.m. but didn't until 3 p.m. Paris was NPO again and not happy. She kept repeating "BaBa" (bottle) over and over, putting her hands on my face to ensure that I was listening to her. I had to continue to ignore the requests and distract her to the best of my ability. She then had two PET scans, and after that we finally had a break from the hospital until February 17, when they would insert a Luke Line for stem cell harvest. She would also get an MRI of the brain and spine. Needless to say I was nervous! I prayed for a clear scan with no new spots. Her counts were coming back, giving her an appetite and energy!

She was eating everything from broccoli and strawberries to mac and cheese and pizza. She went from 6.5 kilos to 6.8 kilos in just five days! Our first antibody treatment (8H9) was scheduled for March 3, followed by scans on the 4th and 5th. The second antibody treatment was scheduled for March 17. Overall, she was doing well. She started to crawl and pull herself up again! She finally had energy to play.

Side effects of chemotherapy often prevent bone marrow from producing white blood cells (WBC), red blood cells (RBC), and platelets. White blood cells fight infection, so without a high white count, you are subject to neutropenia and risk infection. Red blood cells bring oxygen to all parts of the body, so a count below 8.0 tends to cause weakness and fatigue. Platelets help stop open wounds from bleeding. A low platelet count (thrombocytopenia) increases the risk that serious bleeding can occur within the body. Treatment will be discontinued and/or doctors will not perform surgery if the platelet count is below 75.

We started the Granulocyte Colony Stimulating Factor (G-CSF) shot on Friday, February 13. Filgrastim G-CSF (Neupogen) stimulates the formation of blood cells. It helps the body to produce white blood cells after chemotherapy or transplant. It also stimulates neutrophils to prevent infection after chemotherapy. Neupogen aids in stem cell collection. Each G-CSF shot costs approximately $3,650. When giving either G-CSF or GM-CSF shots, other patients have found it beneficial to use an insuflon catheter.

Lucky for me, I lived with so many people at the Ronald McDonald house who had experience with giving the shot, so I asked my friend Aaron to do it for me for the first three days. He showed me how to give the shot step by step. I held her down, and he gave the shot in the thigh muscle. It helped because by him giving her the shot, I didn't look like the bad guy in Paris' eyes. I was the one able to comfort her after it was over.

The doctors wanted to obtain a total of 5 million stem cells from Paris to freeze in case we needed them in the future for transplant. On February 17, they harvested 1.1 million; therefore we had to return to obtain more. Since I had to keep giving her the shot when we arrived back home to Chicago, I decided that I would have to get over my fear and just learn how to do it by myself with no help. This meant holding her down myself and giving the shot with my free hand. At home, I would be 40 minutes from the hospital and alone with Paris, without the luxury of living with so many experienced families battling neuroblastoma.

So one night I rolled up my sleeves and just did it, telling myself over and over that I had to for her health. I was sweating bullets, questioning if I was in the right location, and she was crying and flailing, so that intensified things. She screamed and pleaded with me as I approached her with the sharp needle. I struggled to hold the needle in the right position with one hand as I tried to also hold her down with the other hand. I squeezed her thigh and tried to push in the injection through the skin, but skin is actually tough to puncture. Once the needle penetrated the skin, I pushed the solution through the syringe fast because I was told it burns as it is entering the body. "Mommy no, no…please mommy no!" Paris screaming those words will be forever engraved in my mind. After a few minutes of intense screaming, she was fine. I must say that I did cry, too, after that first time because I felt very bad and guilty about sticking her. I feel bad when others stick her, but I felt worse because this time I was the one who was inflicting pain. The second day I gave her the shot, she twisted her leg and the needle came out before the injection went it, so that day she got stuck twice. I really felt bad about that. I would feel terrible after I gave it to her, but over time I got more comfortable with the process. I even tried to do it when I thought she was in a deep sleep, but as I gently touched her leg, she opened her eyes and stared at me and screamed and I just forced myself to do what I had to do without emotion.

To extract stems cells, Paris' line is hooked up to two tubes on the machine – one to pump white blood cells out where stems cells are produced and the other to replenish the blood with by donor blood. It usually takes a few hours, and she usually sleeps through it. No pain, just a long day. On February 18, we tried to extract more stem cells but only got 800,000. On February 19, we tried again and we got 2.6 million. The grand total collected and frozen were 4.5 million. They initially wanted 5 million but decided that was close enough.

On February 20, we had an appointment to remove the temporary line. We also got the MRI results from Dr. Kramer. She said it looked good and was pleased with the results. She stated that there was enhancement in the sites that had post-operation surgery, but no other areas indicated a tumor. The area resembled what she would expect post-operation surgery enhancement to look like. I was very excited about the results; however I always worried about the microscopic cells and possible active neuroblastoma within the area. But I would worry about that when I had to. At that moment, I had to take the positive information for what it was, that it resembled post-operation enhancement.

I obtained a copy of the report from her MRI brain/spine scan to read for myself. I noticed that the report for the lumbar spine indicated that there was enhancement most likely from post-operation and radiation, as the team had told us; however, it also indicated that there was a discrete 1 x 0.6 centimeter enhancing nodule between T9 and T10. The report stated that the changes extend toward the neural foramen but do not enter the spinal fluid. The impression also stated post-therapeutic and new mild residual paravertebral disease. In regular terms, that meant there was less than a centimeter of disease that they believed was still present in the spinal area, according to the report. The doctors had not mentioned this when we discussed the results of Paris' scans. Perhaps because it was so small, they wanted to wait and see, believing it would disappear on its own. I sent the doctor an email that included the following:

"I am glad to overall hear that the enhancement is only identified in the surgery sites and could be a result of post-operative/radiation but just was concerned when the report identified dimensions and stated mild residual paravertebral disease. Since this scan was compared to the one in January, would I be correct that this nodule was not present before? Paris is scheduled to receive 8H9 in March. Am I correct in thinking that the antibody only affects the spinal fluid/canal? If this is the case and the nodule is located between vertebrae, how will we approach treatment for that area? Would it be possible to intervene with something as she receives antibody? My concern is that eventually that nodule will enter the spinal canal, being that that area is the original tumor site."

Paris weighed 14.74 pounds and was maintaining her weight. Overall she was doing great. The treatment was still on schedule, and we would begin antibody 8H9 on March 3. Hopefully the antibody would attach to any remaining neuroblastoma cells. We were on a week break, only needing to go to the hospital for blood labs/work and medication.

After experiencing New York and the constant travel back and forth between the Ronald McDonald House and the hospital, I found it necessary to purchase a stroller that would accompany Paris with ease. I researched a lot of jogging strollers and decided to purchase a BOB jogging stroller with front-wheel rotation. This somewhat expensive stroller is very reliable, and I was able to write it off on my taxes because I used it for a medical purpose. The stroller is capable of reclining and can carry up to 80 pounds, which is perfect for transporting children to and from the hospital after a procedure or treatment after sedation.

We attended St. Catherine's Church in New York on 68th and 1st Avenue when we were staying there. The church is in the same direction as the hospital, so we would always stop in either before or after our day at the hospital. Whenever Ralph, Paris, and I went together, Ralph would hold onto his host and then break it in half for Paris to eat in the church pew. Since Paris had not yet received the sacrament of communion, she was technically only to be blessed and not receive the body of Christ. But we figured that she had been through so much that we were sure God would overlook that sin. Since she had obtained the body of Christ once, she felt entitled to receive it every time.

One time, Paris and I were in New York without Ralph and attended mass. During the communion procession, I carried Paris up to obtain the body of Christ. She is observant and started to hold out her hands like everyone else, and as we walked toward the priest, he proceeded to bless her. He gave me the host in my mouth since I was holding Paris, and my intent was to quickly take it out of my mouth and then break a part of it off to give to her, but by the time I got back to the pew it had melted! When we sat down, she called out, "Mommy, where's my piece? He didn't give me my piece! I want my piece!" I tried to explain that he needed to get more and that we would have to get some tomorrow, and she continued to call out, "But mommy, he's giving more to them," as she saw other people receive it. She cried, repeating with her loudest voice that she wanted it and that it wasn't fair. Needless to say, when we went the next day, I just ended up giving her the entire host because I felt so bad about the day before.

The day finally came for Paris to receive her first antibody treatment. In March, she began receiving 8H9, which is tagged with radiation and only travels within the cranial/spinal fluid to target any microscopic neuroblastoma cells that may remain. She would only receive 8H9 a total of four times. On March 3, Paris received what was considered a test dose of 2mCi. Over the next two days, the team tapped her Ommaya to drain and test Paris' cranial/spinal fluid. The PET scan followed to ensure the flow of the antibody. It showed that the antibody engulfed the entire area to ideally surround and attack any remaining cancer cells.

She received her second dose on March 10. This dose was much stronger, at 34 mCi, and classified her as radioactive. We had to spend the night in isolation in another hotel room. The following two days, she received a cranial/spinal tap to check the fluid and test the level of radioactivity. I was under strict orders for this dose. An average adult is only allowed 500 m rem per year. Paris was giving off 190 m rem per hour, meaning that if I held her, I would reach my legal limit within three hours. The team recommended that I keep a distance of three feet from Paris and a distance of six feet from other children and women who are pregnant. They told me that I must limit holding Paris to 30 minutes over those three days. If necessary I could hold her more, I would just be over my limit.

Well, you know I broke the rule. How could I not hold her when she was screaming? I thought after everything she had gone through, I could handle a little radiation. We did find humor where we could, though. One day while she was radioactive, she actually set off the alarm at the pharmacy. I was wondering why every time I walked in and out of the store the alarm would go off. After sharing the story with a friend later, she helped me make the connection.

As the days passed, she became less radioactive, and she tolerated the treatment very well. Her favorite word was no, especially to me when it was time for medicine. She would cover her mouth and fight me 'til the end. She talked a lot, blew kisses, and gave high fives. She had started to pull herself up onto objects again, so I was hoping that in a few months she would be walking and running all around. Elmo and Barney were now tied as her favorite characters. Her hair was starting to come back, and again it was totally different than the first two times. In the front it was blond with little frizzes, and in the back it was straight and black.

Assuming that her scans continued to look the same without significant changes, she would finish the last two doses of 8H9 – which would be another test dose and then a larger dose – on April 7 and 15. She would then start on the other antibody, 3F8, which targets cells outside the cranial/spinal fluid. After as many as 14 rounds of that, she would start an oral chemo, Temodar, for one year. I couldn't even imagine how that would go. We were on it for five days, and it was a nightmare! I'd have to teach her to swallow, with M&Ms or Tic Tacs, so she could take pill form instead of the liquid.

As always, things can change in a second based upon scans. Our next MRI of the brain and spine was scheduled for April 1. If the spot on the last scan, which was attributed to post-surgery/radiation, were to change in the scan on April 1, we would need to figure out a plan to treat that. I hoped and prayed that the spot remained the same and we could continue on with the plan.

Chapter 15: More Antibody 8H9

On April 2, I received the results from the MRI of Paris' spine. They revealed that the enhancement areas remained the same, and one spot actually became smaller in size without treatment. The antibody 8H9 that Paris received did not affect these areas outside the spinal cranial fluid. They again resembled enhancement from post-surgery and/or radiation, less likely from disease. The team continued to monitor those sites closely.

I was still waiting on the results from the brain MRI, but as it is often said around here, no news is good news, so I hoped that that would be the case for us.

The antibody 8H9 that Paris received targets the cranial/spinal fluid, which hopefully would give us good results in the brain area. Her platelets were low, dropping from 40 to 24 in just a few days. This could have been from the 8H9 treatment or because she had a bit of a cold, which could suppress her immune system. Platelets determine if antibody 8H9 can continue because it is linked with radiation. The platelets would need to recover on their own, otherwise she would have to switch to antibody IV 3F8, which does not contain radiation and targets everything outside the cranial/spinal fluid. This type of antibody is much more painful than 8H9. It was on our list of treatment, so this meant we would be doing it earlier than planned. The final dose of 8H9 would be put on hold until her platelets recovered.

This trip was by far the most complicated, just because I must have changed my flight at least 100 times. I'm sure Jet Blue got tired of my calls! They were kind enough to credit my flights as I shared my story with them. In the past, other airlines have not been as workable, as they have hidden policies regarding flight insurance, which has caused me to lose a lot of money. For example, in this situation I had to change a flight due to a scan scheduling. The travel insurance paperwork states to contact the airline. I asked to change my flight, and based on the fact that I had travel insurance, the flight should be switched without a fee. However the insurance package that I purchased specifically stated in the fine print that "preexisting conditions" do not allow for a reimbursement in change of travel plans.

I thought that being on the 8H9 antibody would be very easy, and my stay in New York would only be two weeks to receive the last two doses of antibody treatment, however, again things had changed. Paris' platelets were extremely low. When we began treatment, they were 200, and they had since dropped to 15. Since they were below 50, the criteria for children with a CNS relapse, we could not continue. We would have to save the last two doses for the future (hopefully we will never need them).

The results of the brain MRI were stable compared to February. There was no evidence of disease, and the area resembled post-therapeutic change from surgery and radiation. No news was good news.

The results of the spine MRI compared to February showed the areas of enhancement between T10 and T 11 were no longer present. Paris still had the spot on T9, which remained stable in size (1.0 x 0.6 centimeters). It was hard to determine if the spot was disease or post-therapeutic change. Since it was stable, I hoped and prayed no disease, but the location was so close to entering the spinal fluid as time went on. The plan was to begin antibody IV 3F8 as soon as possible to prevent that.

This is the story of how Paris had a terrible, horrible, no good, very bad day.

There is a lot of "work up" and necessary steps that need to be taken before the start of IV 3F8. Paris began that on Thursday, April 9, and was NPO, so we already had started the day off on a "great foot." We went to clinic and had blood draws, and she needed to have an NG tube placed for contrast for the CT scan. She threw up the first dose of contrast and had to be re-dosed. Then they had to take a four-hour urine sample, where a catheter was placed, so the day was really bad now. The saddest part of the day was when she was screaming "Help me, help me" and "Mama, no...no...no." Of course she held her urine, plus she was NPO for the full six hours, and we only got a little sample! She needed an Echo scan, which showed fluid around her heart (which is a bit scary because heart damage is a possibility if one has had a lot of chemotherapy). Those results led to us having an EKG scan to track her heartbeats. After that, she was sedated for bone marrow testing on four sites, which is extremely painful. Since her platelets were so low, she bled all over from the bone marrow aspirations and wouldn't stop, so my tan shirt became soaked in red and she needed a platelet transfusion. Needless to say I began to panic! After all that, we needed to do another blood draw to ensure that the platelets took and discovered that we needed a blood transfusion because she lost so much blood!

There was one more important test that needs to be completed, which is the two-day MIBG injection and scan. The first day consists of the nuclear medicine injection, where Paris would become radioactive. On the second day, she would receive the actual scan. We were waiting for an opening to do that scan, which would give us more information about any other possible disease that hopefully is not present.

I had to stay in New York until all of the workup was complete, and everything was processed to begin IV 3F8. Once we started IV 3F8, it would only be every month for five days.

Again all of this was contingent on her health, counts and scans. Everything can always change in a heartbeat...

There was the swine flu outbreak in April/May of 2009, and everyone was getting vaccinated. The swine flu (H1N1) versus the regular flu vaccine was a big debate for us, being that Paris had not received any of her vaccinations except for the first dose of hepatitis B because she was diagnosed at such an early age. As long as the flu virus was not an active/live virus, Paris was allowed to get it. The H1N1 vaccine came in both the live (nasal spray form) and the inactive (shot form). We then questioned if we should get the vaccine for both the regular flu vaccine and the H1N1 for fear that if we were to be exposed to the live virus, Paris could be at risk. Ralph and I both work in schools and have exposure to many germs and would feel horrible if we were to have caught something and expose Paris to it without her having the vaccine. We decided that Paris would receive both the regular flu vaccine and the non-active H1N1 shot, and Ralph and I would receive the regular flu shot.

People caring for children with cancer must be conscious of some factors where vaccinations are involved. Receiving the live/active virus contained in vaccinations can potentially do damage to our children who are in treatment, as their bodies are immunosuppressed and not able to fight off any type of germs. Individuals who have not been vaccinated may have a deadly effect on the very children that we are trying so hard to keep healthy.

It is important to recognize whether the virus contained within the specific vaccination is "live" or "dead." Consider getting the shot, which is a "dead or killed" virus, as a way to prevent the flu. Live viruses, which are given as a preventative measure for children and adults in hopes not to obtain the flu, can spread and be passed into the immune system of a compromised child. It is not recommended for children in active treatment or who have recently completed transplant to be given the vaccine for regular flu or swine flu in addition to any other vaccines because they are immune compromised.

On April 22, I would be leaving New York for 10 days. Before I left, the team prepared us for our next treatment plan, IV 3F8. I heard it is quite painful and there could be a lot of unexpected complications that accompany it, therefore Ralph would be traveling with me. I was worried about the process, as everyone going through it the first time should be. The doctor stated that the antibody IV 3F8 has no long-term effects, and in Paris' case, being that she is so young, she won't remember the incident. My husband made some good points as well that we were doing it for her as a needed treatment. By no means does any sane parent want to inflict pain onto their child. Ralph said that in order to build a beautiful city, you need to tear down a few walls. I agreed that it was for the good of the cause.

Everyone keeps saying that there's a reason for the pain that I am enduring and that I just can't see that reason right now. That it's not meant for me to know at this moment. I believe that there are reasons for everything. I just wish that it would be brought to my attention soon, because it is so hard to continue on and not have answers to why. If I had justification, such as we are going through this because our child will be the one that brings a cure to this horrible disease, then maybe I could accept it better. What is Paris' role in all of this? Why was her soul chosen to be put through so much pain? Why was my soul chosen to be her mother, to watch someone I love suffer so much?

There is a poem that is written by Terri Banish entitled, "I Still Would Have Chosen You."

> If before you were born, I could have gone to heaven and saw all the beautiful souls, I still would have chosen you.
> If God had told me, "This soul would one day need extra care and needs," I still would have chosen you.
> If He had told me, "This soul may make your heart bleed," I still would have chosen you.
> If He had told me, "This soul would make you question the depth of your faith," I still would have chosen you.
> If He had told me, "This soul would make tears flow from your eyes that could fill a river," I still would have chosen you.

If He had told me, "This soul may one day make you witness overbearing suffering," I still would have chosen you.
If He had told me, "All that you know to be normal would drastically change," I still would have chosen you.

Chapter 16: My Relationship

Neuroblastoma is designed to break people apart. To fall in love with someone is easy, but to stay together during a crisis is extremely hard work. When presented with this type of situation, it becomes a real test of character and a test of relationships. You either are able to make it through the situation, and it brings you closer in some sort of strange way, or the stress can break you apart, changing your relationship forever. I have seen partners stick together more than ever, with the traumatic event ultimately bringing them closer together, and I have also seen it destroy normalcy within a relationship, causing people to separate.

The average relationship requires work to keep it afloat. Fighting with your spouse is normal to a certain degree. Every relationship has a degree of arguing that is considered healthy. We all know that men and women are different in the way we think, interpret messages, act, and display our emotions. It's challenging enough to sustain a relationship and learn each other's habits and personalities without incorporating children into the mix. When children enter the relationship, they naturally increase the stress level between partners.

Relationships require even more work when you add a sick child into the equation. Get ready to experience stress at an all-time high, especially when it's time for any type of treatment or surgery. We heard messages differently, saw situations differently, expected different outcomes, and dealt with things differently. Ralph's way of handling things is by simply shutting down when they get too overwhelming for him. He knows his limit, and I am working on finding mine. His body allows him to take a break and enjoy life, but mine won't until business is done. That's something that I need to work on. Not only did we disagree about everyday things, but we then had the added component of a life-threatening illness, medical care, and responsibilities. At times the situation became very stressful, and the threat of divorce slowly replaced the words I love you.

My mother and father divorced, and I was raised in a single-parent household. I told myself that was the last thing I would ever want for my child. Before Paris was born, as every couple does, we had our ups and downs but always worked everything out. Then we found out that Paris had cancer. One would think times of crisis would bring couples closer together, but there were times that I experienced the opposite. I would never wish this situation on anyone, but I was so upset that it happened to me. The possibility of cancer never entered my mind, even though I knew it affected children. The severity of it just doesn't register when you're not in that situation. I was so upset all the time, blaming so many different things, even Ralph. I was resentful that he had three healthy kids from previous relationships, and here we had the ideal situation and I get dealt an extreme circumstance. I felt like he didn't understand me at all. Remember, he has a half-full personality, so where he was trying to see the positive in things, I would interpret that as he did not understand and was not sympathetic.

When we were away from Ralph for treatments, I felt like a single mother, being by myself and having my family split. I give so much respect to families who are caring for their child as a single parent while managing multiple children.

Ralph and I had even more fights during our journey, but ultimately we needed each other through it. We both needed to really dig deep into our souls to remember what brought us together and realize that we each play a vital role in our relationship and balance each other quite nicely. I really do believe that having both of us together helped Paris through this. She has seen us argue, but she also has seen us make up and be each other's support. She has seen love from both of us, and she always is the center of both of our attention.

I must give my husband a lot of credit for being able to fly independently to New York, live there alone at the Ronald McDonald house, make medical decisions, and take care of Paris. Many partners, when faced with this situation at some point, decide that caring for their child with cancer is too much to handle and choose to walk away. I have seen so many wonderful women forced to care for their sick child – in addition to other children they have – without any help. It's a life-altering change, and these women conquer it. They are able to get up each day and perform the most respected obligation alone. I feel very blessed that I have a partner who has been willing to face every challenge with me. Being a parent of a child with neuroblastoma, you face your ups and downs, most of the time more downs, and search for the positive during it all.

Neuroblastoma causes the dynamics in the household to change. I thought that we would be a 50–50 partnership with Paris on a full-time basis and that she would want us equally. But she has seen me play a significant role in her life and wants me constantly. This led Ralph to feeling unwanted, unloved, and not needed. She calls out for me, wants me to hold her, and wants me around all of the time. She favors me as a parent, which is not how I saw our parenting strategies. I also thought that we would do things together all of the time and share the responsibilities equally, but I have become the sole caretaker of Paris and he has become the provider of the household.

He would find out what was happening secondhand and was unable to be there physically. It must be very difficult to be in a house when no one is there because they are away for lengths at a time. It must be very lonely to come home to an empty house when you had expected it to be filled with so much joy and happiness. Ralph also wanted the opportunity to help raise his daughter since his other children did not live with him. He was robbed of that opportunity for the first two years of Paris' life.

Chapter 17: Antibody 3F8

Prior to beginning the antibody treatment, Paris was assessed by the team. She now weighed 8.1 kilos, or 17.8 pounds. She also grew to 28 1/2 inches; however, she had what was thought to be a right leg length discrepancy. Her right leg was 1 inch longer than the left due to the severe curve in her spine caused by the tumor impact. This could be modified with a shoe lift on the left foot, which orthopedics had made. That helped her to walk/run all around because she was finally balanced.

We returned to New York on May 3 for the first round of IV 3F8 antibody treatment. Neuroblastoma is seen as part of the body, and therefore the immune system or white blood cells do not attack it naturally because they see those "bad" cells as normal. The IV 3F8 antibody is derived from mice, so those antibodies overstimulate the white blood cells to become better fighters of foreign objects within the body, being the cancer. The targeted antibody carries a marker to attach themselves onto the floating or remaining neuroblastoma cells. The white blood cells are stimulated by daily injections of Granulocyte Macrophage Colony Stimulating Factors (GM-CSF) and see those marked antibody cells as foreign. Since they are attached to the neuroblastoma cells, the white blood cells attack them.

I had prepared myself for the worst pain that Paris would have to endure. Paris began IV 3F8 to target any microscopic or remaining tumor neuroblastoma cells within the body. This treatment was scheduled for five days out of the month. The doctors want to get at least four rounds in, assuming she doesn't become human antimouse antibody (HAMA) positive beforehand.

HAMA measures how strongly the body's immune system is reacting to the 3F8 antibody. It is a sign that the body is developing a response against neuroblastoma. Once a patient develops HAMA, 3F8 antibody treatment is no longer effective, as the HAMA blocks 3F8 from reaching the neuroblastoma cells. The patient undergoes blood tests to determine if he or she has become HAMA positive or negative approximately two weeks in between treatments.

It's very difficult because as a parent, you are told that you want the child to experience pain when the antibody is administered because that indicates it is working.

So at 9 a.m. we began the first day of the 3F8 antibody experience. This is said to be the most difficult because the nurses need to figure out how much dilaudid – a specific pain medication used when dealing with antibody 3F8 – to dose her with, as they tailor it specifically to each child. There is a fine line in determining how much each child can handle because every child is different. It was trial and error. They first gave her too much, and her breathing slowed down to a scary pace. The team feared it would stop all together, so they needed to reverse it with naloxone chloride (Narcan), which counteracts the effects of narcotics. Waiting for the reverse effects to occur, doctors came in and began shaking her to wake her up because she was in such a deep sleep and her breathing rate was slow. As I sat and watched her lay still and lifeless, I immediately thought that she died.

Once they tailored the correct amount of dilaudid, the antibody continued to flow through her IV. Almost immediately I saw a reaction. Paris exhibited pain by grunting, and I could feel her stomach cramp and tighten. She became red and sweaty and cried out in pain. It was difficult to see this. I asked the doctor if Paris was experiencing the most pain possible and then wondered about the context regarding what I had said. What parent asks if their child is having pain because they want them to? The children in the rooms next to us screamed and moaned in pain. There is a certified music therapist who, during the process of 3F8, plays soothing music, trying to divert the children's attention to music and massage while they are experiencing excruciating pain that lasts two hours. Paris then remained severely uncomfortable for another three to four hours. I began to wonder why I was doing this to Paris – reminding or convincing myself that it was for the best.

Hearing Paris scream, "Mommy No!" with endless tears and look of ungodly fear as she is approached by anyone wearing scrubs or a white medical coat will stay with me. It's such a conflicting message for a child. We have to do harmful things to help her get better. I envisioned her always laughing and happy, planning a wonderful life for her. She has had limited exposure to a carefree life. And I have been robbed of the infant stage with her, which I wanted so badly. I have no idea what it's like to have a baby from 0 to 18 months old. I missed all of the milestones. I have one milestone from the hospital; constantly overcoming obstacles.

After the infusion, she was given pain medication to relax her, which caused her to sleep for hours afterwards. Some children get rashes or hives, but Paris did not exhibit these during the infusion or afterward. By 9:00 p.m., she woke up almost as if nothing happened and was back to normal. Little did she know she would start the same routine again for the next four days.

Days 2, 3, and 4 of antibody 3F8 were challenging, as Paris' heart rate was noted as very slow, or it would beat an extra beat, like a gallop, which was concerning, therefore they put her on 24-hour watch. The team determined that there could be a few reasons for this. It could be because the Medi-port placement had shifted, adding pressure to the heart, meaning that they may need to surgically remove the port, causing a delay in treatment. The stress of the antibody could cause an irregular heartbeat, or the worst-case scenario, Paris may have developed the initial stage of heart complications from prior chemotherapy treatment.

I hoped that treatment would not be postponed and she would not become HAMA positive after round 1. The overall plan was to complete four rounds by August and then begin 10 months of Temodar in combination with Accutane. It is said that Temodar has no harsh effects like the other chemo treatments, so we could ideally have a "normal" life again. Not a bad plan if things could stay on track.

With just one day left of Paris' first round of antibody treatment, continued heart complications gave us a one-way ticket to the ICU for more tests. Stuck in New York AGAIN! They decided to remove Paris' Medi-port to see if the catheter impacted the heartbeats, but it didn't and now Paris is stuck getting all her infusions through an IV.

I was very nervous to learn the outcome of further heart testing. Upon discharge, the team determined that it was a benign complication, but when triggered by the antibody it could make the situation much worse. They recommended that I follow up with the cardiologist in Chicago and obtain monitoring and an EKG.

These follow-up tests showed that the port was not causing the problem. A normal resting heart beats between 60 to 100 beats per minute. The cardiologist determined that Paris has frequent atrial ectopy from an unknown etiology. She has periods of bradycardia related to blocked premature atrial contractions (PAC) and had a Holter to monitor the skipped, paused, or irregular beats.

Chapter 18: And Just Like That, It's Over

We were scheduled to start the second round of IV 3F8 at the beginning of June, however we ran into a delay. During her first round, Paris only received two days worth of antibody rather than the full five days when they sent her to the ICU for her irregular heartbeat and removed her Medi-port.

I assumed everything was on track, and Paris and I flew to New York. When we got there, they stuck her twice trying to get the IV and then said they were going to delay treatment. I was in shock because I had just spent the night before throwing up and mentally preparing myself for the second round of IV 3F8. I was still trying to figure out how this happened. My conclusion was that either the EKG from Chicago was not sent at all, it was sent late and the team in New York didn't have time to review it, or the team in New York didn't read it until I arrived and had yet to devise a plan. I could have stayed home for a few additional weeks. So now I was here for nothing and just waiting until they figured something out.

They said that with her continued irregular heartbeat and the stress and medication of IV 3F8 that if the right people are not in place during the antibody treatment two things could potentially happen: the first being fatality and second her oxygen level could drop so severely that it could cause brain damage. Both of these possibilities were not a pleasurable option for me. It was obvious that they wanted to be prepared or possibly stop treatment all together. They stated that they would be more comfortable doing treatment across the street at another hospital where there was an ICU floor in the event that something happened, but it would be difficult to transport the antibody. They worked to figure out the next step or plan of action that is best to take. We had to just wait for them to come to a decision.

When the cardiologist consulted with me, she seemed extremely worried, which was different from the average "this could happen" discussion. She went on to discuss possible medications to control the irregular heartbeat or inserting a pacemaker. I couldn't believe my little girl might need a pacemaker. My grandfather, who was in his 80s, had a pacemaker. Is this really the discussion we were having? What changed from three weeks ago when the condition was still present?! You really never know what news to expect when you enter the hospital. What a way to start. I should have known better – nothing in New York is easy. I was just trying to believe that everything happens for a reason and even though it was a bump in the road, maybe it was supposed to happen this way.

While we waited for the team's decision, I thought about the options. First, I thought we should do a PET scan to determine exactly how much disease, if any, was left. Maybe that would answer our questions and she would not need the IV 3F8 now. Maybe we would get that other dose of 8H9 that we missed or maybe we would start oral chemotherapy now. The good news was that the neuroblastoma vaccine was ready at Sloan-Kettering and had been approved by the FDA. I hoped she would qualify to receive it. Good things are constantly being developed at Sloan-Kettering, so hopefully the next finding would be that cure.

The team analyzed the results of all the heart monitoring, and Paris was diagnosed with premature atrial contractions, meaning she had regular-irregular heartbeats. Basically it meant that sometimes there would be irregular beats present and other times her heart would beat normally for many beats without interruption. She could have been born with it, it could have been caused by treatment at 10 days old or it could have occurred over time from her cancer treatments. It made no sense to go back and try to figure out how or when it occurred. Going back to analyze the how's and why's would only waste valuable time that we needed to figure out how to handle this and how it affects treatment options.

The team concluded through EKG scans that irregular beats were present, but when the onset of antibody treatment occurred, the irregular beats became more frequent. Basically, you had a precursor, and when provoked by the antibody treatment, it got worse. Her heart rate became very high and her oxygen level dropped very low, which was a dangerous combination. Therefore, they discontinued IV 3F8 and deemed that the risk outweighed the benefit.

Antibody treatment is an experimental clinical trial, therefore we don't know if it is the "save all." There is no guarantee that after receiving antibody that neuroblastoma will never return. Some children have done wonderfully after receiving the antibody as a component of their treatment plan, but others have relapsed. I wish that there was a guarantee, but there's not. So based on the facts, I had to think very hard about what was being presented. I had to put so much mental and physical effort quickly to cover all of the possibilities because we were dealing with the life of my child, and I couldn't afford not to ask questions or research other options that may or may not be presented.

I was alone on this trip. It was extremely difficult making decisions alone and trying to figure things out in a day and trying to have very serious conversations over webcam or on a cell phone. Ralph and I understood that Paris had neuroblastoma, but above all she was Paris first, and we valued any treatment plan as long as it didn't sacrifice her quality of life. We understood that everything has risks. We will never know if our decision was the right one, but it felt like the right one at the moment. Sometimes you just know as a mother. I just couldn't take a risk that has the numbers and evidence to support the two very devastating outcomes. Who knows if she could have tolerated it just fine, but at what expense am I willing to try it? I know Paris' personality, and I would never take that away from her. I would rather lose the battle to cancer than to rob her of her personality. If you ever met Paris, you would agree that she is not Paris without it. Without the daughter that I know and love, I really wouldn't have her anyway. I would just have her body, and I consider that selfish on my part.

I guess the most important thing is to always remember that you cannot second guess yourself. Once you made your decision – that's it. There is no turning back, no should haves, no could haves, no would haves and no regrets.

I once heard "Never take any progress for granted. Every milestone met, no matter what timing, will be cause for a celebration."

It took us 18 months to get to the IV 3F8 treatment, and just like that we were no longer able to continue it.

I wanted to at least get the four cycles, which is said to be the safe zone. We only received a total of four days, not even the full five-day dose. It was very disheartening because it took so long to finally get to the antibody stage, and it was so quickly taken away. I felt like this was what we needed and now. I felt like our options just worsened within a day, but I then had to refocus. I had to look at the situation differently, and just like that, I was thinking about why Paris shouldn't get treatment. The rules of this game are not fair. There are no choices that provide the perfect answers. The options are all are horrible in some way, shape or form, so basically you are just choosing the option with the lesser of the two evils. It was a disappointment at first to learn that we were not able to receive the treatment that Sloan was noted for and that everyone desired to receive, but maybe it was a blessing in disguise for us.

On June 4, 2009, we started giving Paris 75mg/m2/day of Temodar for 42 days, which is a standard treatment for brain tumors in children and adults. When we left New York, the plan was to place Paris on five cycles – 42 days on with a one-week break and then repeat for 10 months, which is equivalent to 210 days. There is a pharmacy called Cherry's that can compound the Temodar into liquid syrup, making it easier for an 18 month old to take. It will also add almost any flavor.

It's like being at 31 Flavors; however the most popular flavor to mask the chemo taste is grape or chocolate. We selected grape.

Overall, she tolerated it well. We gave her the dose in the morning, and then we went about our day. At first, it was tricky to decide whether to give it with or without food, at morning or at night, but after a few trials and errors, we figured it out. We always gave Zofran first and had a bowl and napkins ready, just in case the chemo came back up. If Paris could keep the chemo down for at least 25 minutes, it was in her the system and we didn't have to re-dose even if she threw up later. But if she threw up instantaneously or before 20 minutes, we had to re-dose to ensure the dose was given. Each bottle of Temodar is approximately $1,400 and contains a certain amount of doses. Therefore if Paris threw up a dose, there was limited extra. Cherry's Pharmacy provided me with a stopper system at the top of the bottle so that it was easier and cleaner for the syringe to pull out the exact amount without having to worry about spillage.

Everyone is always nervous before giving medication, let alone a toxin like oral chemotherapy. There is no right way to administer it. It is important to keep your composure, and it really is trial and error. We usually taste her medications to see what she is experiencing. Ralph decided that he would also taste the Temodar, which is toxic, before giving it to her. I couldn't believe that he would actually taste it knowing that he doesn't have cancer. Ralph gave the medicine to her daily. He has made comments that if something long-term happens, he would feel horrible because he administered it. I questioned the long-term side effects of giving Temodar for 10 months straight. It is one of the only chemotherapies that cross the blood brain barrier, which caused me to think that Paris' little developing brain was receiving a low dose of chemo daily. What will be the effects of that in the next few years? Two-thirds of childhood cancer patients will have long-lasting chronic conditions from treatment. The medical staff can't give definite answers about the long-term side effects because there is not enough research. Paris will be a contributing factor to provide data for future kids. Hopefully this will not adversely affect her. I struggle with the decisions we make for her at times because quality of life is important to us, but I ultimately don't want another brain tumor to arise. You really walk a fine line between treating the disease now and not knowing the outcome and life afterward.

As I walked down the streets of Manhattan, specifically 5th and 6th Avenues, I looked around and thought to myself, this is a very strange scenario. In New York, people walk around with high-end shopping bags possibly containing a single shirt or a purse that may cost $1,400 alone, and I was walking around with a little bottle of chemotherapy!

"You will encounter people who will restore your faith in humanity."
The Truth 365

Every once in a while, you meet someone who really makes you examine your life. I often wonder why I meet certain people at specific times and why they entered my life. When I was in New York, I had a lot of experiences that I believe have sent me signs, messages, or interventions when I was at my worst. Out of the blue, a stranger would stop me and say, "What a beautiful little baby. What's her name?" I told them, and they would go on about how she reminds them of someone or how they had a grandchild around the same age. Once they saw her hair, they would ask what was wrong, and I would tell them the story. They would always finish with, "I will keep her in my prayers tonight."

People commonly stared at Paris, both when she looked like a cancer patient, with no hair and thin, as well as when she resembled a healthy, age-appropriate child. People seem to lock into her eyes. I often hear how gorgeous, pretty, beautiful she is from total strangers that just feel the need to comment. If I had a dollar for every time I heard a comment regarding her physical appearance, I would be rich. It was always in New York that I felt things happened for a reason. I felt like when I was in New York, I always came across a person that I was destined to meet. People there came into my life at random times, just when I needed them. I always felt like I received mini messages that always left me thinking, "That was very strange that such and such just happened."

On one of our trips to New York, on the subway, a woman stopped us to tell me what a beautiful baby Paris was. She locked eyes with Paris, and it gave me the feeling right away that she felt something different about her. She began to have tears in her eyes as she was stating how lovely she was. She engaged in a conversation with Paris for a while, and I got the sense that she was very heartfelt about the brief interaction. Something drew her to Paris. I began to think about this incident. Was this a stranger that was simply drawn to a child, or was there more to it? My mind began to race as I tried to dissect what was happening. Possibly she was a woman who couldn't have a child at all and was drawn to what she couldn't have. Possibly she was a woman who may have at one point had a child that resembled Paris and she felt a connection. Possibly she was an instrument from God and was acting as one of his angels to send a message to Paris from someone in heaven who wanted to meet her or speak to her through this woman. The instant connection was too strong for me to just ignore. Then, just like that, she got off the train and we departed, but I felt that Paris had left an impact on this woman.

Sometimes when people commented on how cute Paris was, they would notice that her shoe looked a little different and ask what happened. I would comment that she was in physical therapy. At times, surprisingly, some people said their child was also in physical therapy and reassured me that she would be fine after about a year or two of services. I would think to myself, "If it were only that easy...having just PT as your only problem." At that point, I would tell them that it was more complicated than that and that she had cancer. They would not know what to say, and then the next most infamous question was, "It's curable, right?"

My response to that it would be, "Well, it's cancer and it's unpredictable."

In the hospital cafeteria one day, I ran into the gentleman who conducted Paris' radiation, and we began talking. He stated how big and cute she had gotten, as he remembered her from when she was an infant. The gentleman serving the food overheard our conversation, and after I had placed my order, he gave me a voucher so we didn't have to pay for our meal. Kind actions like that happened all of the time while in New York.

A gentleman at the Belaire Building in New York gave us the imagining disk of the many x-ray images that were taken of Paris' spine that I needed to bring back with me to Chicago. When I asked how much a copy of the disk was, he stated, "Regularly it would cost $50, but today it's free."

I met the strangest people at the strangest times who said the strangest things. Out of the blue, I met a woman who asked me about my computer. As I told her about the pros and cons about the computer, we began a conversation and she quickly learned about Paris, her diagnosis, and how we ended up in New York. After listening to Paris' story, she approached her stop on the subway. Before she left, she wanted to re-iterate to me that she will remember my story and pray for Paris. She left by saying, "When you think that I forgot, remember that I'm praying for you."

There were a few newspaper articles written about Paris since her diagnosis because her case is unique. It never ceases to amaze me that there are people who will either go out of their way to help you tremendously or to hurt you when you are already down. I went to my mailbox a few days after an article about Paris' journey and upcoming fundraisers was published. I opened a letter that was addressed to me. My mood quickly changed as I read the letter. It was a hate letter and I was addressed as an "N" lover. I was in shock. I couldn't believe that someone actually read Paris' newspaper article and took the time to seek out my address and send me this hateful letter. I often think that if everyone spent their efforts and time doing beneficial things, the world would be a much better place. People will apparently go to the extreme to voice their opinions when they feel you are wrong. It was 2009, and there were still families teaching the cycle of hate. Even though I received a hate letter, it actually was a blessing in disguise. Many good things came as a result of it. So whoever sent it, thank you, in a strange way because as you were trying to inflict evil and pain, good actually came of it.

The police officer who responded to the complaint asked if we had any known enemies or had a thought of who would send such a hateful letter. We explained Paris' diagnosis and showed him the newspaper article, which had a picture of Paris with both of us. The picture provided a visual to people who obviously were against interracial relationships, which was most likely the trigger of the letter. The police officer turned to us and asked, "What type of cancer she was diagnosed with?" When we responded neuroblastoma, he nearly turned white in the face. He shared that his 56-year-old sister was just diagnosed with neuroblastoma a few weeks ago and was in the beginning stages of treatment. I gave the police officer information about the disease and hospitals that specialized in neuroblastoma outside of Chicago.

Alissa Groeninger wrote that article about Paris for the *Daily Herald*. Sharing the story about how my husband's students were so dedicated and motivated to donate to our daughter's cause was so touching to me. His students come from very limited backgrounds, so when they were donating change and money that they truly needed to survive, it really was sincere. They went above and beyond by taking a single theme, "Pennies for Paris," and turned it into a life-long lesson. They went door to door selling candy bars. They donated money that they had worked for and bypassed buying shoes for them to invest in the life of another. These acts were truly unselfish. I wanted to recognize them in a positive way. I decided to call every newspaper that I could think of, and out of all of the ones I contacted, one responded. There is a reason why the *Daily Herald* responded, which led to the article being distributed to certain suburban areas, which led to me receiving the hate letter, but it also led us to Donna, who happened to be an author herself and offered to do a book signing fundraiser for Paris. When I analyze it, it seems that everything happened in the order in which it was meant to. Things fell into place even though I didn't see it at first. Then, after a few events occurred, I could piece it together and see that every event needed to happen for the next to occur.

If I look hard enough, I can find the good buried underneath the bad. Many positive caring letters followed the article that focused on support and prayers, which outweighed the single bad one that I received. I believe there is a reason for everything. I didn't know why I was a victim of a hate letter at that moment, but in time I was able to see that it was meant to be so that other things could occur. It was an order of events that allowed me to help others and allowed others to help me.

Chapter 19: Strangers' Acts of Kindness

By July, Paris and I had been home for 42 days. We enjoyed every minute of it and were keeping so busy that I somewhat forgot we were still dealing with neuroblastoma. But all good things must come to an end, and we were headed back to New York for scans at the end of the month. We needed everyone to keep their fingers crossed and offer lots of prayers for a positive outcome so that we could continue to enjoy every day without the constant medical stressors.

When I was in New York, people would always ask, "So how long are you here for?"

I always responded, "It depends on the scans, but we are supposed to leave on…." I always planned on leaving on my scheduled departure day but also knew that I had the potential to stay longer at any time.

Paris was at the age where she was mimicking our every word. I asked Ralph if he had given Paris her chemo yet. Out of the blue, I heard this little squeaky voice call out, "My chemo yet?" It really was a shock to hear. I didn't know how to react, but after I processed it, I thought to myself how sad it was to hear my 21 month old repeat and question if she had received her chemo.

During those 42 days, we went for weekly blood counts. Her counts never dropped, which meant she didn't need any transfusions, she never got sick, and her hair stayed in place. The only side effect was severe mood swings at times. She would range from being irritable, moody, inconsolable, and bossy. When I explained to Ralph about Paris' behaviors, he responded, "So have you been sipping on the Temodar with her?"

We enjoyed trips to the city to go to the aquarium, museums, parks, play dates, and physical therapy, which Paris loved since we went three times a week. Paris was still not walking, but getting there.

Maybe by her second birthday she would be running around. She was really getting bigger, determined, strong-willed, and talkative. We kept busy playing catch up as well with medical decisions, such as the option for medication to regulate her heart to receive 3F8, combining chemotherapies such as Temodar and Accutane, and overall insurance coverage, denials for treatments, insurance appeals – the ongoing story of my life.

There was so much work to do, and I felt like we were always facing a time constraint. I was constantly researching new treatments, faxing, checking emails, matching bills with Explanation of Benefits (EOBs), and talking to people on the phone, writing letters, or working some problem out. In July 2009, Sloan-Kettering announced two new treatment options that would be available should we ever need them. I also attended the two-day neuroblastoma conference in Chicago and obtained so much more information there. It was very good, but it was definitely information overload. I sometimes felt like I was neglecting Paris' need for attention just to get her what she needed to give her a chance at survival.

Time is always a constraint. There just isn't enough time in the day, and there is only one of you, so when you combine your odds, a lot of things can't get done.

I felt like I had been robbed of me. I used to be energetic and organized and had everything pre-planned with a back-up plan. I felt trapped. I felt like I would never get out. I felt like it was so unfair. I felt like sometimes I was crazy because one day I would be fine and then all of a sudden, out of the blue, I would break down, questioning again why this had happened to me, even though I knew I wouldn't get an answer. Then, after my long hard cry, I would just get up and keep on going. It's like I needed to release a build up before I could move forward with the ongoing tasks and mental and physical exhaustion. Sometimes when you have no energy or strength for yourself, you don't realize you are actually someone else's strength.

I had a running list of countless things, and just when I thought I got ahead, something else would pop up that put me back at square one. My mind was constantly racing. Sometimes I would be working on numerous tasks at a time, and honestly I was functioning on a very thin rope that was holding me together.

People asked me when did I have time, how did I get it all done? The answer is I feel like I don't have time for anything but the medical aspect of this. I forced myself to stay awake until 2 a.m. to try and catch up. I tried to stay one step ahead, but I always felt like I was sinking. The normal thing to do is to take breaks and know your limit, but I was so used to pushing myself and not let things hang over my head. My motto was what I can get done today, don't put off until tomorrow. At times there was limited time for fun with Paris, no time with my husband, and definitely no time for me. The key is you have to stop and make time and go out of your way to make time for the important things because the medical aspect will be there forever. It will always be a constant component of your life.

We began our second 42-day cycle of Temodar on July 23, 2009, and it started off well. I hoped it would continue to go well. We were scheduled to go back to New York from July 26 to 31 for scans. Every day we had something scheduled. The days consisted of MRI of brain and spine, CT, MIBG, PET, urine collection, and bone marrow aspirations. I was able to really analyze the process while in nuclear medicine as we awaited Paris' MIBG injection, which contains a radioactive isotope. I watched the nursing staff bring up the isotope in a sealed container sent via Fed Ex from New Jersey. They began to put on gloves, masks, goggles, and coats to protect themselves from touching the harmful toxic substance. The same substance that they are so careful with had been injected into Paris every three months as part of her routine care.

I am proud of the medical accomplishments that Paris has made over her first 20 months. I am so proud of her for drinking 7 of the 8 ounces of contrast for her CT scan. I am proud of the fact that she is still a true fighter and has become a self advocate when medical personal try to examine her.

A few days before leaving for New York I became so overwhelmed with feeling like I couldn't do it anymore. I was constantly battling with insurance, appeals, and feelings of anxiety with Paris' upcoming scan results. It's conflicting when your child looks so good but you feel something horrible is growing inside of them. So I basically crumbled into the fetal position on the floor and began crying for a while. I couldn't control it – the feelings of sadness poured out. The next day, my mother's friend at work, who just happens to specialize in organizing medical bills and appealing claims and bills that have been denied, gave me her number. I attribute it to a divine intervention that came just when I needed it to relieve some of the burden and stress that I had been feeling, especially with organizing medical bills, since I had thousands of explanation of benefits for more than $2 million worth of services at this point.

Chapter 20: Ralph's Turn in New York

The airport used to be very stressful for me. At first, I always went with someone, and then I had to start making the trip alone. I would always have to go through the special security because I had enough liquid medications to be questioned. I had a stroller, car seat, diaper bag, travel swing that was attached to the stroller with a bungee cord, my carry-on bag with all of her distractions for the plane ride, and a purse. Picture that as I walked through the airport. Not a lot of people offered to help me. They wanted to cut me in line and looked as if I was in their way. My glances back relayed the message – like I really wanted to travel alone with an infant, not to mention a sick infant, who requires all this crap. Sometimes I would wish that Paris would just puke on the person sitting next to me who saw me struggling in the security line and did nothing to help, but she was always a great plane rider. I could read people's facial expressions as we walked down the aisle, which clearly indicated that they hoped we didn't plop down next to them. As we sat down next to that lucky person, they would always ask if she has traveled before. My response was always the same. "We do this every month. She likes the plane better than the car."

We arrived in New York without a problem and settled in, seeing too many familiar faces. It was good to see everyone again. I just wish it wasn't at the Ronald McDonald House or at the hospital.

On July 27, we went to clinic, and Paris had to get stuck eight times before they found the right vein for an IV placement. Since the removal of Paris' Medi-port, every procedure required an IV stick. IV placements were very difficult because Paris would fight very hard and her veins were small, which caused them to blow out. I honestly miss the port. The port made every stick so much easier because she didn't feel the needle; she simply fought the anticipation of the unknown. Now she was older, verbal, and stronger, and her cries were that much louder. Holding her down was very difficult, and it would usually take five people to try to get it on the first try without blowing out any veins. After every IV stick, Paris demanded a bandage, and as her lips quivered and tears ran endlessly down her face, she looked for confirmation by saying, "I'm so brave, right mommy?"

I of course confirm that she is brave, the bravest person I know.

After she calmed down a bit, Paris would want to call her daddy. When Ralph answered the phone, I could hear her say, "Daddy I just got an IV, and I was so brave," sniffling between words.

On Monday the 27th, we had the brain MRI and echo. Tuesday was the PET injection, PET scan, and MIBG injection. Wednesday was the MIBG scan and bone marrow aspirations. Thursday was the CT contrast, which I was able to get her to drink the entire 7 ounces only after two hours of playing tea party using lemonade-flavored crystal light. That last day of scans also included a CT scan, MRI of the spine, and 24-hour Holter to monitor the heart.

We flew home from New York on Friday and got the phone call early regarding the scan results. The brain MRI was clear and showed no evidence of disease! The PET, MRI of the spine and CT showed uptake and increased growth of 1 to 2 millimeters on T9 that had previously been stable since January. The plan was to complete the second cycle of Temodar until September 2, return to New York for a CT scan and compare the results. A biopsy would follow, and most likely she would undergo surgery number four with Dr. LaQuaglia to remove the mass.

On August 26, 2009, I began my school year. I was at work when I learned of a child I personally knew who had passed away from neuroblastoma. I instantaneously felt surrounded by death. This was the first child that I had connected with. A child with cancer, other than my daughter, who I personally knew. I saw this child on certain days in horrific pain and then on other days extremely happy. I saw him being tutored for school. I had conversations with him, and now I learned that he had passed. The typical phrase one hears is that the child lost his battle with neuroblastoma after a long fight. Realistically it's an unfair battle, one that no one asked to be part of. Is it fair to say he lost something that he had absolutely no control of? The fight and battle that was not fair to begin with? To say he lost seems so unfair. I believe he didn't lose. He was unfairly taken by the disease, stripped of his strength, and robbed of his ability to fight.

I knew when I woke up the morning of August 31 that I would have to deal with a very difficult transition later that day, after my work day had ended. My mind told me that I wanted to rush home to spend as much time as I could with Paris before she left, but my body kept finding things for me to do at work because subconsciously I knew that as soon as I got home, reality would set in. Paris would leave to go to New York with Ralph, and I would stay behind. Needless to say, August 31, 2009, was one of the hardest days for me. It was the first time that I would ever be away from my baby since she was born. I had been the one that traveled with her since she was diagnosed. My role was to take care of her and be there for her every moment. I drove them to the airport and watched them as they passed through security, disappearing into the crowd, and then I left the airport alone. I drove back home alone. I sat in my house alone. I ate dinner alone, with no noise and no one to take care of, no one calling for mama, and finally, I went to sleep alone. I missed Paris terribly. What do I do when my sole purpose is gone? I consumed my time by calling Ralph nonstop, reminding him of every little detail that I could think of, and when I wasn't calling him, I cried, wondering how I was going to survive without her for the entire month.

I tried to do other things to relax myself or preoccupy my time while she was away, but then when the day was over, I was faced with the reality that I was all alone, and I couldn't help but think about what was really happening. I wondered if she missed her bedroom with all of her belongings, how horrible it must be for my daughter to understand that she can't read all of her books at bedtime and be limited to the five that she brought with her. That she can't play with all of her toys at leisure, can't swing on her play set outside, and that she needs to adapt to the change in environment.

I stayed alone in my house for a total of five weeks without my daughter. My husband solely cared for her in New York while I worked to maintain our insurance coverage. I worked not because my heart was invested in my job, not for the socialization, not for the money, but solely for the insurance. How do you explain to your child why you can't be with them? She would ask, "Where's mommy?"

Ralph would respond, "Mommy's at work."

Paris would then say, "I miss my mommy." Work was the last place that I wanted to be, but I was forced to be there to give her the best health and medical care I could.

It's a shame when you begin to debate which is more important; a paycheck or insurance coverage. I would choose insurance. It is sad when you have to weigh spending time with your child who is sick or going to work to provide necessary care for her. I can't get those moments back, and I ended up missing a ton of milestones and important things all because I had to work so that in the long run she would have the care she needed to grant her the possibility of a long life full of health. I find myself always making choices, and none of them are good, which comes down to making choices based on which of the evils can I live with and which I can't.

I missed her so much and cried every time I heard her little voice on the telephone. I couldn't help but wonder is this a strange way for preparing me to be alone without her? As I spoke to Paris over the telephone, she wanted to give me a kiss. She said, "Mommy, I kiss the phone." How sad is that that you are forced to be apart from your child for months at a time and give kisses over the phone, and she can only hear your voice and not be physically around you? I would always ask Ralph to show her my picture so she doesn't forget me.

As I would hang up, I would look around my house where all of her toys are perfectly arranged, just like she left them. I didn't go into any room of the house except my bedroom. I almost felt like I was living in a museum, where everything is just properly placed and there is no life within the house. I was missing every aspect of her. I was missing seeing the things she does. I wondered if when she returned to me she would be different because I would have missed over a month of her life.

The roles were now reversed for Ralph and me. When I was in New York with Paris for the longest stay of three consistent months, I now knew what Ralph was feeling and what he meant by both sides of the coin are hard. It is difficult for the parent who is with her to consistently manage her medical issues and take care of her needs alone; however, the parent who is at home alone is also in a difficult position, managing the necessities of the household alone and not having her around, in addition to trying to cope with this situation from afar. When I was in New York alone, I would call Ralph and ask what he was doing. He was always doing things to keep busy and take his mind away from sitting in isolation and being confined to one room of the house. I interpreted that as "having fun" while I was struggling to care for Paris alone. But once I was forced to be home, I was the one trying to keep busy. When I returned from New York, I got upset. I wanted and expected the house to be perfect and spotless because I figured he had nothing but time on his hands. But being on the reverse side of this situation, I didn't even have the desire or energy to enter another room other than my bedroom, and cleaning was the last thing on my mind. This experience has given me a new perspective on how Ralph felt when I was away with Paris.

Ralph tried to comfort me by saying that at this age, if you're "outta sight, you're outta mind." He would, however, say that Paris would ask about me every morning when she woke up but then continue on her day fine without me. As time went on, would she just accept that I'm not around? I wondered if she would have a stronger bond with Ralph, wanting him over me when something was wrong. Would she remember me? Would she be upset with me for not being there? Would she forget about me and be distant, or when she returns, would she see me as a stranger? Or would she return to normal and act as if I was never away?

I missed my husband, but honestly, it seemed that when we talked, more insecurities were present because there was a fear that we were drifting apart due to a constant separation. In everyday situations, the more and longer people are separated, the more they tend to lose that daily connection, especially if there is a huge stressor forcing it. You wonder what the other is doing. You lack communication, patience, and quality time, and you lose sight of each other because you're focusing primarily on your child. It takes a tremendous amount of work and energy to maintain a normal marriage, so imagine the effort, energy, and other factors needed to keep one together with a child who needs treatment, on top of that out-of-state treatment.

I would occupy myself by going to work, but I really didn't feel like I had a purpose. My sole purpose was in New York. I questioned what I was doing, why wasn't I with her? I was held back. I had to work to keep insurance. It has been estimated that even with insurance coverage, the average family will have an out-of-pocket expense of about $40,000 per year, not including travel. I couldn't visit as often as I would like because I had to reserve my sick days. I felt like no matter how hard I tried to make things okay or tolerable, something else would pop up, whether it was bad news, something I had to do with insurance, nonstop phone calls, daycare arrangements. My mind was always asking questions and researching treatment options. I felt consumed by these thoughts, and it seemed for every one to-do that I checked off, another was right behind.

I hear that I'm strong all of the time, but sometimes I just want to be weak. Am I really strong? Am I strong when I am crying nonstop because I can't see my child for more than a month? Am I strong when I can't see my husband for more than a month? Am I strong when I have to work and do a job that my heart isn't really invested in anymore because my daughter consumes my thoughts and time? Am I strong when I look at other children and wonder why Paris has to suffer through so much pain? Am I strong when I have to repeat the same story from the beginning to people who ask? Am I strong when I'm afraid every time they take her to surgery or treat her with harsh toxins? Am I strong when I question my faith and have to try to pull the positives out of a negative situation? Am I strong when finances are tight and we are struggling to settle a debt that we didn't even create? Sometimes I question what it is to be strong…and sometimes strong wasn't me.

During my pregnancy I would have ongoing thoughts about the future revolving around what I was going to do and not going to do as a parent, things that I was going to teach her, do with her, enroll her in, and expose her to. I thought I had everything outlined and planned and that I was pretty prepared to be a mother to my daughter. Little did I know that life isn't set in stone, and it throws you curve balls along the way. Never in a million years would I think that I would be faced with the most ultimate challenge after just having her.

Chapter 21: Paris' Fourth Surgery

I felt like I was in a constant whirlwind for the past two years. Every September thus far, we had begun treatment, and then things slowed down in January. We would have a less complicated three-to-six-month period, and then we would go for scans and end up right back where we started.

I think about how at one point Dr. LaQuaglia was a young boy. He and his parents did not know that their son would grow up to be a world-renowned surgeon, saving other people's children. I think about his talent and the gifts he was given to save children's lives every day. Can you imagine being that person, going to work and saving lives? Parents pass him their children, believing in his confidence, skill, and gift to remove a tumor that no other surgeon could. I was one of those parents that handed my child over to him, putting nothing but trust in his surgical plan. He takes no credit for his work and whole-heartedly believes that he is only an instrument guided by God. He feels he was placed on Earth for a purpose, and people benefit from his work, saving lives every day. I am honored to be in his presence.

We met with Dr. LaQuaglia on September 8, prior to Paris' fourth major surgery. People live their entire life and do not experience surgeries or anything this drastic, but she was only 22 months and already going through her fourth. We entered Dr. LaQuaglia's office and greeted each other. We immediately let him know that we are glad that of all people we were seeing him again. His response was grateful but reminds us that seeing him is not a good thing. It subconsciously became a normal routine before every surgery. I became sick to my stomach, I would get severe cramps. I was unable to eat, became fatigued, and tended to throw up and have diarrhea. I was an emotional wreck before, during, and then a few days after surgery, until Paris was back on her feet.

Dr. LaQuaglia never says that he performs miracles. He has operated on many children, and I feel a sense of relief when he takes them under his wing. He stated once that he thinks of the mothers of these children, and his main goal and primary focus other than to remove the entire tumor is to get them back to their mothers. He blesses his hands at St. Catherine's Church in New York before every single operation. He states that only God can perform miracles, but he has been given a gift to act as God's hands during the countless hours that these children are under surgery.

Ralph and I sat with Dr. LaQuaglia and heard about the potential risks of surgery. We mentally prepared ourselves for the necessary conversation of informing us of all of the tragic, horrible things that could occur during the procedure. The list of what could happen went on and on. We listened attentively, but by this time we basically had it memorized. We knew that the spot located on vertebrae T9 was about 1.6 millimeters and that it was the only spot of concern.

We felt confident beyond words with our surgeon and that this surgery would be alright compared to the three previous experiences. We learned that the removal of the mass would take approximately two hours. However, at this point Ralph and I knew better than to ask or require a time period because we know his response would be "as long as it takes for me to do the job right." He goes above and beyond, searching the area for additional suspicious spots, and works so diligently when removing masses in such difficult locations.

In discussing the dimensions of the mass compared to what it was in the previous months, Dr. LaQuaglia logged onto the computer and retrieved the images from the previous months. As he discussed that area, he began to discuss the plan of removal for the other area. Ralph and I looked at each other in shock. Another area? At that moment, we learned that Dr. LaQuaglia was planning to remove two spots rather than just the one that we were informed of. Ralph and I were dumbfounded. We had to backtrack at that moment because we were completely confused. No one had ever told us that there was an additional spot in question. We didn't even know it existed. Apparently, there was another mass located about 2 centimeters below vertebrae T9, by the vena cava that he also planned on removing. After Ralph and I got our bearings back, we focused on that spot as well and now were discussing the two spots that he was planning to remove.

Our immediate concern was the communication among the oncology team. The surgeon is just instructed to remove the masses. The team didn't inform us of the second mass, which really made it difficult for Ralph and I to mentally prepare and have a conversation regarding our daughter when the surgeon knew more than we did. We were supposed to be on the same playing field and have the exact same information. It also made us look uninformed that we didn't even know the exact treatment that she was supposed to be receiving the day before it was to occur. We should not have been blindsided.

When you meet with a surgeon, it's a very scary thing to begin with because they are basically holding the life of your child in the palms of their hands. Ralph and I tried to ready ourselves for the discussions and have all of our questions and concerns written down, but when you come face to face with the surgeon, your mind loses track of everything. All I saw was the man who would be taking care of my child the following day. To look someone in the face and realize that they would be performing a miracle, an act that not anyone can do, to potentially take the disease out, is mindboggling. How can someone's eyes be trained so well to focus on those tiny cells that are causing so much damage? I was struck with amazement and sincere appreciation accompanied with great fear all at the same time.

He continued to ask if we had any questions along the way, but we didn't. It really comes down to this being necessary. If we didn't do it, she would die. The only question that was really important to me was, "If it was your child, you would do the surgery, right?"

His response was yes, and he felt confident that he could remove it. That's all Ralph and I needed to hear. It was a manageable spot in a very difficult location. We were giving her the best chance at life as well as focusing on the quality of life she would have. There really was no other option.

On September 10, 2009, Ralph and I passed Paris off to the surgery team for the fourth time. It was always difficult. It never seemed easier, no matter how many times we passed her off. By now, we should be familiar with this process, but it always seemed like the first time when you pass your child off to a team of strangers and hope and pray for the best possible outcome. They took Paris, and it was two hours before they even entered the operating room. Then it was another two hours before they even made the first incision. So we just sat and waited.

As I waited, many thoughts would cross my mind. I'd think about what children will become later in their lives, what is their purpose. I think about Dr. LaQuaglia and Dr. Cheung from Memorial Sloan-Kettering, and I wonder how many mothers were hoping that someone like them would eventually come along to save their child. They were now here for my child, and I was so thankful. Dr. Cheung said once, "There will be someone smarter than me in the years to come." I wonder who it will be. Maybe a survivor? Maybe Paris?

God watched over Paris yet again during this surgery. She went in at 6:30 a.m., the first incision was made at 9:45 a.m., and the surgery was completed at 12:30 p.m. It went very well, and we again were blessed with the best possible outcome. During a previous surgery, when Dr. LaQuaglia came out of surgery, we heard the words, "The mass appeared to be neuroblastoma." This time he approached us in the conference room and said it resembled more of what appeared to be treated neuroblastoma and explained the difference. He said that the mass located by T9 appeared to be capsulated and seemed to be firm rather than the typical neuroblastoma formation, which tends to ooze out and separate when trying to remove.

He also removed the spot by the vena cava and biopsied it. He commented, "You know, I've been doing this a long time, and it looks like a mature form of neuroblastoma called ganglioneuroblastoma, but the microscope will be the final judge and the pathology will be confirmed on Monday." I felt like I could take a breath again, at least until Monday when the pathology results came in, which would determine our plan of action. Ralph and I sat with her in the ICU, waiting for her to regain her energy, and I kept whispering to her how strong she was and how proud I was of her.

After while, Paris looked up at me with her puffy eyes from the surgery and said quietly, "Mama, I go home now?" What do I even say to that?

I told her soon and reassured her that mama and dada were here with her.

I sat for hours stroking her hair and holding her hand. These were the times she needed me. She expected me to be there and to make the situation better. These were the times I felt powerless and helpless, but I needed to be strong so she didn't see it. She could only see me as strong – tears needed to come in private, not on her time.

This time, Paris was able to verbalize that she was in pain. She said right after surgery, "My mama" in a quivery voice, and it broke my heart to hear her say, "Ouchie, it hurts mama, it hurts so bad." She spent at least three hours recovering in a holding room and was then transported to an inpatient room. Her only little request when she realized that we would be moving was that she wanted to hold my hand the entire time during the transport from floor to floor.

We thought she would sleep a few hours and rest, but not Paris. Within 30 minutes of getting out of surgery, she continued to ask for her bottle, and then after countless requests started to demand it. "Mama, go get it now!" and "My baba!" We had to wait until her stomach made noise again and "woke up" after surgery. She's got a lot of fight in her. After four hours of sitting and waiting to get a bed in the Pediatric Observation Unit (POU), she woke up and looked us straight in the eye and said, "I want to go bye bye." It just broke my heart because I wanted to scoop her up and take her away to a place where she wouldn't have to experience any pain at all.

Staying inpatient is kind of like jail. You don't see the outside world. You are confined to the hospital room, and you don't notice anything else around you. You know that you have been in the hospital awhile when you are inpatient and you call the hospital food good. I had to catch myself and reevaluate what I said. I thought to myself, did I really just say that hospital food is good?! Am I really evaluating different floors' and different recovering rooms' food menus? Oh my God, what is happening to me?! That was what it had come down to: evaluation of hospital food and actually thinking it was decent.

I received an email from a fellow neuroblastoma parent where she compiled a list of things that indicated that you had been fighting neuroblastoma way too long.

Here were some of my favorites:
- When you're at what is considered a "normal" procedure and the doctor advises that general anesthesia will be required and you are not even bothered.
- When your child has pneumonia and you hope it's an oncolytic virus because that's the kind that kills neuroblastoma cells.
- When another child throws up in public and you're the first to clean it up without flinching.
- When your child complains of something hurting and you hope it's a broken bone.
- When EMLA cream is regularly carried in your purse.
- When kids with hair start to look strange to you.
- When you can sleep anywhere and in anything that reclines 15 degrees.

- When you're not surprised when your child is holding a conversation with the doctor in specific medical terms.
- When your child won't let you touch anything in a public restroom.
- When you're best friends with the pharmacist.
- When your know more about the nurse's personal life compared to your own family members.

Surprisingly, Paris was discharged three days after having surgery, and I was very happy to see that she was so resilient. I was also surprised to hear, as we packed her into the stroller, her demand that we go to the park across the street from the hospital and swing. This view is torture for kids who are in treatment – looking out the window and seeing other kids having fun. But, it can also be a reward for them when they are finished for the day. Ralph and I thought to ourselves that swinging may not be a very good idea due to the surgery site, but as we walked by it, she screamed even louder, "I swing mama!" So her little wish was granted, and we went to the park on 68th and 1st. This park is ridiculous. There are four infant swings and a long line of mothers and caretakers waiting to put their child on the swing. Ralph and I pushed Paris, and she laughed. I saw her strength as she swung. She just wanted to be a kid without any restrictions, limitations, or hurt. Apparently, nannies in New York have a known, unspoken rule that you have a five-minute limit and then you must let another person have a turn. I felt a few glares as we obviously exceeded our "time limit." I can handle the stares, but if anyone would have made a verbal comment, I would have definitely said, "If you only knew that this little girl just had surgery and all she wanted to do when she left the hospital after three days of laying in bed was to come to this park and swing her little heart out, maybe the glares would stop."

Ralph's brother called me, and we began talking about Paris and her prognosis. I shared with him her persistent character of wanting to go to the park and swing literally just after we got discharged from the hospital. I was sharing a funny story about Paris' persistent nature when he asked me, "What does that mean to you?" Without giving me a chance to think about it and answer, he responded for me by saying, "That she has a drive and that her character is strong. She wants to live and is going to live – you can't go anywhere but up from here."

I left Paris with Ralph on September 13, 2009, as she slept in her crib at the Ronald McDonald House recovering from surgery. I never thought that I would ever leave her without saying goodbye. I told her I loved her while she was sleeping. As I walked toward the elevator alone and out of the front door toward 73rd Street where I would catch my taxi, I felt an unbearable amount of guilt and sadness. I began to question if I was doing the right thing by leaving her. I was in such a dilemma because I knew I had to return to work since I could only take 14 days off during the new school year, and I had already used four in the first week. I had to plan not like a mother would, but strategically, which meant thinking with my brain and not my heart. I knew I needed to save those days in the event that I needed them. I wondered if she would wake up missing me, calling for me, and I couldn't be there. I had to remind myself that Ralph was there with her, and she has an equally special bond with him and would be fine.

Paris' surgery/pathology results showed that the spot by the vena cava was benign (no cancer), which is great news. It was considered ganglioneuroblastoma, meaning that the cells have responded to treatment and are present in their most mature form but still require more treatment. This is far better than receiving an active neuroblastoma diagnosis/pathology. Ganglio comes in two forms: ganglioneuroblastoma (mature cells that have been treated) and ganglioneuroma (benign neuroblastoma). We were right in the middle between neuroblastoma and ganglioneuroma. That was considered to be fifty percent on our way to being hopefully cancer free. The team would meet to devise a treatment plan. I thought they might choose radiation on the spot if the area falls outside where she was last radiated, and from what they were saying, low-dose chemo, most likely irinotecan. I asked about high dose, and they said most likely not due to the size of the tumor and shape that was removed, but the decisions were yet to be finalized.

Chapter 22: Faith

"When it rains, it pours but you have to remember to look out for the rainbow, because without rain, you would never see some of the most beautiful rainbows." -unknown

"You will question your faith, find it, or renew it." -unknown

When I think about this, I try to remind myself that things happen for a reason, even though I have no idea what the reason is. I believe that there is a great plan for Paris' life. For someone to have to go through so much there has to be. She has brought countless people together, made people value what they have – their health and what they are blessed with, treasuring the basic gifts such as walking, hearing, and speaking because when faced cancer, those things are not guaranteed. Cancer forced me to see the simple pleasures of life, believing in miracles, and it forced me to test my strength.

"Be not afraid, only believe. The body doesn't lead the person, the spirit does." – unknown

I can honestly say that I feel watched over by Father Rookey, a healing priest. In the past when I was going through everything and everything was very new, I called and he picked up every time. I spoke to him, and he prayed for Paris. As we moved forward in our journey, there were times when I felt the need to call Father Rookey, but I was not able to get through. When I tried to call and request prayers during Paris' interim scans, it was very difficult to reach him. But, when I was sitting in clinic with Paris on October 4 during our MRI, I got the urge to call. His secretary picked up on the second ring, and I requested a prayer for Paris that day. I feel as if they know when Paris needs intervention prayers and when she will be okay.

People always tell me, "I'll pray for you." I believe in the power of prayer and that miracles can occur. Paris has been on countless prayer lists, and her name has traveled to places all over the world. I received emails from people I don't even know who are following her story. God undoubtedly has plans for Paris. I've come to understand that I can't ask Him to change this situation; rather I have to ask to understand why it is occurring and to grant me the strength to face it.

"God grant me the serenity to accept the things I cannot change; courage to change the things I can and the wisdom to know the difference." The Serenity Prayer

People's theories vary on why things happen to them. I personally believe that everything happens for a reason, and events in our lives are meant to happen, some of which have been pre-planned during the creation of our souls. I feel that we are carrying out events that are meant for us to experience, and we determine which path or route to take that will ultimately lead us to the next planned or destined event in our lives. I think back on previous people that I have met and wonder why they came into my life at that moment and then somehow reappear during a specific time that I needed them. Or I have met people at certain times that just happen to fit with the situation that I am going through. It feels like people or events just fall into place.

Whatever path you choose takes you in a certain direction. Situations occur to teach you lessons that are intended for you. If you reflect on your life, you may see that you have surrounded yourself with individuals or certain partners that taught you lessons that may be needed for future lessons or to prepare you for situations that may arise in your future experiences.

In my travels, sometimes I speak to the people sitting near me on planes and sometimes I don't. I wonder sometimes, why didn't someone else get the seat next to me, why was it that specific person? It always starts out the same. They say, "Your baby is beautiful...." We get into conversation, and it eventually comes out that she has cancer. I sometimes play a game with myself to see how long the conversation can go before it comes out or when I feel it should come out. One gentleman whom I sat next to was so touched by my story and how we were going to do everything within our power to provide her with the care that she needed that he wanted to help and donate. A stranger; who makes me think about things – was I supposed to meet him on that airplane at that time?

I have randomly stumbled upon people at a needed point in my life. I found myself questioning this as very strange. For example, when I was thinking about writing this book, I met three different authors focusing on cancer-related stories. Was it coincidental or was it supposed to be?

There have been a lot of situations that occurred that should have taken her life already, but it wasn't her time. God was not ready to take her from us. We are keeping her around through the use of modern technology and modern medicine, hopefully long enough for researchers to find a permanent solution and cure for neuroblastoma. We realized that Paris was on borrowed time and cheated death many times. We felt lucky and blessed as she approached the age of two. We were told that she might not make it through the first round of chemo and that after her relapse, we would be lucky to see her reach the age of two.

It never fails. I always receive a divine intervention through random people off the streets of New York. Never before have people been so vocal and forthright when approaching us. There are thousands of people walking the streets of New York, and so many times strangers will approach us and say the most random things that to us are so significant. They will always end their conversation with, "God Bless," or "You have a very special child." I guess you never know who God's angels are among us.

Chapter 23: A Bit of Normalcy

Ralph and Paris got home from New York on October 8 after being gone for a month and a half. Needless to say, I spent most of my time with them once they returned. I must say that Ralph did a wonderful job with Paris in New York. I'm glad that he was able to experience that time with her and deal with the crazy life of nonstop.

The plan for Paris was to be off for three weeks to recover from irinotecan. Then on October 26, she would begin her third cycle of Temodar. Assuming I could keep her out of the hospital and healthy, we would re-scan either at the end of December or early January. I kept my fingers crossed. As of September 10, 2009, she was officially declared as No Evidence of Disease (NED). I just prayed that this would continue for awhile, if not forever. Live one day at a time.

She was also starting physical therapy again that week. She remembered Lisa and couldn't wait to see her again. I hoped her walking would improve and come to her more naturally. Surgery set us back a bit, so we were starting from square one again. She was taking 13 to 20 steps independently, so I was very happy about that. We would continue to work on it.

On October 13, 2009, I dropped Paris off for her first day of daycare, and it was actually better than I expected. I was very anxious the night before because Paris would have to be exposed to a new situation again. She went without a problem. Ralph reminded me that this was what I had wanted to experience – the normal worries in life. This was the time when I should be excited that we were finally able to experience the dropping off at daycare and picking her up after work since it had been two years nonstop of being in and out of the hospital and not doing anything normally. I decided to create my own reality and think positively that morning. I almost didn't know how to handle the typical worries that people have since I had experienced the extreme.

At work, I parked my car as normal and began my teaching day. At about 11 a.m., my principal entered my room and asked me to step outside to talk. He told me that my parked car had been hit by a school bus. Everyone knew that I was happy about returning to normalcy, so I immediately thought that he was joking. Unfortunately, I was wrong. I was parked in between two other coworkers, and everyone who heard about the accident said the same thing, "Out of all people, why did it have to be Lauren's car? Hasn't she been through enough? She's supposed to be on a break from everything and not dealing with these types of things." I reflected on these comments and focused on the fact that with a bus full of students, no one was hurt, which was the first blessing. It wasn't a hit and run, so we were able to handle it through insurance, which was the second blessing. Then I began to think to myself, I'm experiencing normal. Normal people have to deal with these types of things, so I'll take it without complaint.

On October 26 Paris began cycle 3 of Temodar, and she threw up constantly at daycare. She had not previously reacted to the maintenance chemo, but on the other hand, she did have a month and a half break of no treatment, so I thought her body might have to get used to it again. Her body took the medication as a shock and reacted. I thought to myself, "Remember Lauren, its poison that she's taking." The word poison just kept haunting me. It made me realize I was actually giving my baby poison, and her little body had to get used to it. That was absolutely horrific that I as a parent I had to coach myself to say that to put a little ease on the reality of what I had to do. Some combinations for antinausea drugs that Sloan-Kettering suggested were Zyprexa, given one day before, during, and one day following chemotherapy, in addition to Zofran, Ativan, and Vistaril.

On a positive note, that year we actually got to buy a costume at the store for Halloween rather than have one donated to us at the hospital. It was a wonderful moment! It's very surreal how the annual Halloween shopping could mean so much to us. It really does bring tears to my eyes to think that we had overcome a challenge. She was able to put on a costume, God willing, and walk up and down our block just for her to experience it and us to witness it.

I hear all of the time that my family is amazing, which is a very huge compliment, but if you were faced with this situation, you would be amazing, too. You make it happen because you don't have a choice. You give everything you have, make every sacrifice, and/or sell everything you have to provide for your child. I would sell my house and cars and go broke to live at the Ronald McDonald House if that's what it took for her to be healthy.

People mention and share with me the issues that they have and how hard their problems seem to be, but in the midst of their conversation, they see that my expression is somewhat confused, like, "Are you really telling me about the fact that you didn't get any sleep last night because your child had an ear infection?" They turn and say, "Then I think of you, and your story inspired me to keep going, to stay strong and hopeful," or "Your story has put a new perspective on things for me." At these moments I have to remember Ash Beckham once said, "Hard is not relative, hard is just hard." I value their comments, and I know that they mean no harm by expressing their hard or by what they are saying, but in my mind I think, "Thanks a lot. That just made me feel real great, that you recognized that your problems weren't that big until you thought of mine and then you were real glad you aren't in my shoes." It's difficult because people don't know what to say to you and are fearful that what they are trying to say will come out wrong and insulting.

The mind is a powerful thing. If the mind continues to harp on negative thoughts on a regular basis, it tends to believe the negative. It is important to remember that the mind does not control you. Never let it take over with negative thoughts. The moment is not your reality even though you may feel consumed. You need to look past the moment, as the moment will pass. It is important to practice the 3:1 ratio: for every negative thought you may have, you need to say at least three positive thoughts to stay focused. With strength and courage we can make it through another day even if it seems impossible.

As Paris' birthday approached, people asked me how old Paris was, and honestly there were times that I couldn't even answer. I would say, "Um, I'm not sure." There was too much going on to keep track of her age. I could easily remember her schedules, appointments, dates of surgeries/treatments, doctor's names and numbers, insurance problems that had to be dealt with by writing appeals, names of medications and doses, but I couldn't focus on the normal, everyday stuff, like what her first food was, her first word, her first milestone. Those precious milestones that I'm supposed to remember, I just can't. Half the time I'm wondering if I was even mentally there for those events.

My daughter can count to 10, say her name, identify her shapes and colors, name all the animals and their sounds, including exotic ones, and sing the alphabet, but she also knows about her Medi-port, tubies, and ouchies. She can say, "I hurt" over and over and there is nothing I can do but push the pain medication rescue dose available to us every 15 minutes. She can also look the nurse right in the face and say, "I don't like it," as they try to give her all types of oral medication. I have to tell her what to expect and what is happening. I let her know that we are going to take a picture for x-rays and scans, that she will get sleepy when it's time to be sedated, that a tight squeeze/hug is coming for blood pressure, and that an ouchie is going to happen when she will get stuck. These are the types of conversations that I have with my daughter more often than not. To listen to your child say these types of things rather than, "I love it," or "I'm having so much fun," makes me feel like I'm not providing her with the opportunities that I'm supposed to. In my mind, she is supposed to be running around, going on play dates, going to daycare, experiencing the pain of teething, or falling from her first steps. Enjoying life by simply being a kid.

On November 21, 2009, Paris was able to enjoy her second birthday. When I think about her second birthday, I keep hearing the haunting voices that told me she would be lucky to make it to 2. The concept of any birthday after the age of 2 would be a blessing repeated in my head, and now we had finally made it to that point.

Paris had her second birthday party at Bounce Town, an indoor bouncy play area. It was expected to be the happiest time for her since we were finally able to be home and celebrate for the first time. Low and behold, the night before Paris complained that she had ouchies. She tugged at her left ear, and I immediately predicted an ear infection. Saturday morning, the day of her party, I took her to the doctor. Sure enough she had a 3 out of 10 ear infection. She didn't really have fun at her party, but at least she got to attend and experience it. She was a trooper, though, and cracked a few smiles here and there throughout the day.

I questioned why she got sick for the first time since September the day before her party that we were all anxiously planning. I quietly scolded myself and said, "If only I had had the party the weekend before, none of this would have happened."

I took it for what it was worth and accepted that she was able to physically attend her second birthday party with a little ear infection, which honestly was the least of our worries. She ate her chocolate cake and was fully satisfied. At the same time, we have been battling treatment since she was 9 days old, so I never had the opportunity to experience anything normal. Things have always been on the side of the extreme for us, and I have learned to deal with those types of life-threatening issues. Those horrific situations had become my normal, as confusing as that may sound. That night after the party, I literally didn't know what to do about the common cold. She had a runny nose and sneezed a lot. I questioned how to handle this every day problem? I waited so long for Paris to be part of the normal everyday life that kids go through and when she finally got there, I truly didn't know how to handle it because I was so used to the extreme. We continued to give her the antibiotic. I gave her a little Tylenol and plugged in the humidifier and watched for a fever. In a few days, she was back to being just a regular, happy kid.

As she opened her presents from her birthday, I noticed that someone had gotten her a doctor's kit with all of the instruments. I was a bit hesitant when I saw her open the gift. I initially didn't want her to have it since she dealt with the real equipment on what seems to be a daily basis. Paris does not like anyone grabbing or holding on to her arm in fear that she will get stuck by a needle. Being that Paris had endured so many IVs, she wouldn't even let a fake tattoo be placed on her arm. I decided that it would be therapeutic for her to role play and understand the equipment in the home environment, in a less stressful situation. As I watched her play, she was able to identify the stethoscope and use its correct name in context with ease. She was able to use the equipment correctly and mimic what the nurses and doctors have told her in the past. She picked up one of her stuffed animals and said, "I'm gonna give you a shot, okay? It's gonna hurt, okay?" When it came time for giving medicine through the play syringe, she said "It's cherry, not grape. I'm a good doctor." For awhile she associated the grape flavor of the oral chemo with everything, not wanting grape Jell-O, popsicles, candy, or juice. Her imaginative play always ended with a bandage, which in her eyes seemed to make things better for that moment.

Paris had enjoyed being home since her surgery in September. Things were wonderful other than our routine daily chemo (Temodar) and routine weekly trips to the hospital for blood draws and infusions. When I asked her how her day went, she would respond, "Today I got my ouchies, and I got a sticker." It was that simple to her, and it had just become a normal part of her life. Compared to everything thus far, I would gladly take the maintenance work.

Home is a wonderful place to be. She had become quite a character. She was talking up a storm and repeating everything. She made us laugh every day. She continued to be bossy and demanding, but we

136

determined that since that was all she really had control of through all of this, she could be as bossy as she wanted. She knew all of her letter names and sounds, numbers 1 to 11, shapes and colors. She had even pretended to be a mommy to her baby doll. She was so helpful around the house. She wanted to clean up and put everything in its proper place. She loved going to daycare and talked about all of her friends. She was getting so big – it was amazing that she had just turned 2.

For the past two years we had been in the hospital for every birthday and holiday. This was the first year that she had been able to enjoy three major holidays at home – Halloween, Thanksgiving and now Christmas.

On December 14, she began her fourth cycle of Temodar. That month we also went back to New York for Paris' three-month scans and workup, which consisted of MRI of brain and spine, CT scan, bone marrow, blood and urine collections, and MIBG scans. The MRI was the main scan, as it specifically examined the areas where tumors were present and that previously had radiation and surgery. Thank God it was scheduled for the first day. We would know results right away, so at least we wouldn't be as worried for the entire week. As always, we hoped for the best and that we could quickly return home to enjoy another three months of calmness, but we prepared for the worst, as it could happen at any time. We just continued to be grateful for the time that we had.

Chapter 24: Remaining Normal

What a way to start 2010! Have you ever wondered what word is the best word in the entire world? To a cancer mother, the best word(s) becomes "no new uptake" or "stable." Those words you hold dear to your heart and hope to hear them after every scan.

We received the news that Paris' MRI, CT, and MIBG scan results were clear and showed NO EVIDENCE OF DISEASE!!! We had the shortest trip to and from New York – a total of just four days! The brain MRI indicated that Paris had a sinus infection, which could easily be taken care of and was the least of our worries. She did very well throughout all of her scans, tests, and bone marrows – a real trooper. We were glad to be back home, where we could return to work, Paris could return to daycare, and overall we could enjoy normal life for another three months. We would return to New York in April for another set of scans. Until then, we would continue to be as normal as possible and enjoy every minute with Paris. She would continue taking Temodar daily until at least March.

On March 14, 2010, Paris finished her fifth and final cycle of Temodar. That meant a total of 210 days of taking grape-flavored chemo – so I was glad for my little baby to get a break from that. It was a wonderful feeling to wake up and know that today would be the last day that we would have to hold her down and anticipate when and what she had eaten to avoid her throwing up the dose. It was a great feeling to know that component wouldn't be in her everyday routine. It was a great feeling to know that her little body could begin to adjust to not receiving poison every day. It was a great day to think that after today she could just be a kid.

We enjoyed three months, from January to April 2010, at home doing normal, everyday things, with the exception of occasional follow-up and routine care. Paris went through some ear infections, strep, and colds, which we gladly dealt with. During our time at home, we learned of some difficult news, as some of our friends along the way had passed, which was especially hard for me to deal with because we were able to be at home. The average age of death for a child with cancer is 8, causing them to lose 69 years of expected life. The death of a child is one of the most traumatic events a family might face.

Paris had gotten so big! It was hard to think we had been doing this for two years straight. April approached quickly, and we headed off to New York once again for our three-month scans. They again, by the grace of God, came back clear, showing no evidence of disease. We went back home, able to enjoy another three months of normalcy. Her hair was getting so long, but I refused to cut it – we had worked too hard for it. I just kept telling her to push it out of her face or I would clip it back for her.

Paris was sick with the "normal" flu, and as I cuddled her, I began to get teary eyed just thinking about everything that she had gone through over time. Now I was actually sitting here comforting her for a normal issue. Paris turned to me and looked me dead in the eye and said in a matter of fact voice, "Mom, stop whining."

She was talking like an adult and turning into a little character. A new treatment plan that just began was the neuroblastoma vaccine that some of our friends were fortunate enough to be part of. Paris could be a candidate for this treatment plan as well if her next set of scans came back clear. Only time would tell. God was in control of that. So we would go on until July and enjoy the days we were given because we knew firsthand how valuable they were.

During those three months, from April to July, we were blessed to be consumed with living within the normal routine of everyday life. We took Paris to Disney World, where she met all of the princesses. After that, she officially thought that she was one of them. No parent in their right mind would ever attempt Disney with a child under 3, as its more work than a vacation, but under the circumstances we decided that we wanted to give her the opportunity since she for the first time was doing well. She said her favorite was Cinderella, but I really think she liked Ariel and Belle, too. We had a great time meeting all of the characters and walking around all of the parks, especially the Magic Kingdom.

At two and a half, Paris continued physical therapy twice a week, which she worked very hard at. I could see her steps improve. She was able to walk around independently. We primarily focused on balance, core/trunk strength, and muscle toning.

One day, Paris' physical therapist was adamant about having her sit with her legs extended in front of her rather than bent like a W. We would always remind her, but she defaulted into the W position, as I'm sure it was easier due to her significant spine curvature. One night, Paris was in her crib and called loudly for me. As I approached Paris, she indicated that she positioned herself into an "Indian style position" all by herself and was so proud!

An orthopedic appointment that summer determined that Paris had a 52 degree curvature in her spine, which is where the tumor originated. We were faced with the decision of whether or not to undergo back surgery to correct the curve. Left untreated, Paris' bones would harden and cause permanent damage as she gets older. The suggested plan was to place growth plates within the spinal cord area to make it flexible as she continues to grow and then consider the placement of a metal rod before the age of 9.

Paris had been off of treatment for neuroblastoma since March 14, 2010. She continued her monthly finger sticks to check her blood work and would receive IV sticks for her Pentamadine infusions until August. At this point we had called the vascular access team (VAT) to place an IV line in the vein before beginning treatment. One day when Paris had her IV and the nurse wasn't putting the bandage on fast enough, she screamed, "Roll it up!" She learned quickly how to express her advocacy skills.

In July, we flew to New York for Paris' routine scans. We were able to enjoy the city a bit this time and did some sightseeing. The team recommended that Paris receive maintenance treatment, which includes low-dose chemo Cytoxan and Rituxan to prevent HAMA from rising and then attempt to receive antibody 3F8 again. It was a very difficult decision to make, as there were many components to consider, such as her heart condition and her immune system, and overall, it is not the "save all" treatment. If you undertreat your child, then your chances of death are high. If you treat or over-treat your child, there is a great chance that she will suffer from long-term effects in the future.

Ralph and I felt that she was finally given a chance to be a normal kid and enjoy life to the fullest; therefore, we decided not to pursue any new treatment at that point and re-scan again in October. If Paris' scans determined there was a need for the treatment rather than just as a preventative measure, we would do whatever was needed in a heartbeat. But at this point in time, we thought that Paris deserved to get a break. We would battle what may come when it comes – if it should come – and know that if there is a recurrence, it was not because we didn't do the treatment. We were aware of the fact that she could relapse at any time and re-enter the harsh world of treatment. We went with our gut, which said it wasn't the right time for us to do this.

Chapter 25: Extended Family

In my experience, friends tend to come and go while on this journey of neuroblastoma. Some friends may start the journey with you and never leave your side; however, some are meant to travel with you for a certain period but not the entire trip. They may start the journey with you and early on may decide it's not where they want to go. Other friends may decide to meet you halfway through the journey. You'll also find comfort in people you never had anything in common with.

Near or far, we are in this together. What affects one affects us all. Countless neuroblastoma families that we have met provided support for us during times of need. We really are there for each other and commonly refer to ourselves as extended family. We listen to each other, console each other and always celebrate with each other. I feel that it is important to branch out to families who are in a similar circumstance. Make friends with them, introduce yourself and make that connection, be an extravert rather that an introvert. When you do that, you can somewhat begin to make sense out of this horrible disease. When you allow yourself to be vulnerable and consult with others in the same boat, just a different seat you allow yourself to heal and realize that you are not the only person who feels, responds, or thinks certain ways.

The reality of this disease is that you can't physically, mentally, or emotionally fight it alone, without the support of others somewhere along the way. I know it gets tiresome repeating the same story over and over, rehashing every detail to people. I know it seems easier to keep to yourself because you're constantly surrounded by families going through the same thing that you are trying to overcome. People in the same situation really do understand, and networking with them creates a sense of comfort. It's nice to know that when the majority of the world doesn't understand why you can't function one day and can the other, when you're crying uncontrollably at the drop of the dime, when you're not able to maintain adult relationships with friends, family, or your spouse, when your mind is so bombarded with so many thoughts that adding just one more will cause you to burst, when you are processing thoughts that no one else in the world would ever think of, when you're making decisions that you never thought you could make and at such a fast pace that you must go with your gut rather than problem solve, when you're giving toxic medication you never thought you would inject into your child just to give them a fighting chance, when you feel like you just can't go on any more – not for another second these same people that you call extended family go through it, they did it, they thought it, and they feel it, too. There's no blame, questions, guilt, or judgment, only comfort and confirmation.

Everyone in the neuroblastoma family is greatly concerned with your child and wants to know how they are doing. They reach out to those in need despite the difficulty in comforting someone else when their own child may not be doing well. I've been in both positions – receiving the good news as well as the bad.

It's so hard to read the many posts and updates about all of the children that you have met on the Caring Bridge sites. It's all too close to home. It's extremely difficult to look at someone else as they are preparing for surgery or routine scans. You never really are safe. We are all a family, and even when it's bad for me, I try to be hopeful for another family.

After being at the Ronald McDonald House for almost six years – living there for a duration of the time and then traveling back every three months – we met so many families, some informally and some we have grown close with over the years.

My friends in the neuroblastoma extended family are wonderful! There are so many people that I have met from all over the United States. I think I can safely say that I know someone from every state. There's nothing but comfort and understanding with this group of people because we are all the same. We all chat about our daily adventure at the hospital and long night ahead of us. We swear that one day the reality show crew will come and document the lives of the women at the Ronald McDonald House titling the show "Real Housewives of the Ronald."

I've been introduced to families who have been newly diagnosed with neuroblastoma and asked to speak to them. It's an honor that people see me as so knowledgeable, but it again is that double-edged sword because no one wants to be an expert on this topic.

When your life becomes engulfed with hospital stays, the staff and doctors who work with your child almost become your extended family. You see them so much, and they know your child almost as well as you do from a medical standpoint. They are working in collaboration with you to save them.

I once commented to a friend who also happens to be a cancer mom, "Don't get me wrong. I love that we are friends and that I have you as a support person, but I hate that we were forced to be friends under the situation that we both faced." I tend to feel like my new network of friends are all cancer moms, and I sometimes wish that I didn't have that network as my dominant group of friends. Sometimes it just overwhelms me to think that I'm surrounded with conversations about therapies and fundraisers on a daily basis because everyone is in the same situation. My main groups of friends that I once had have been forced to become my secondary group of friends because the more time that passes, the less we have in common.

Chapter 26: Can This Really Happen Again?

Since Paris was diagnosed, I have a new respect for the month of September. September is national cancer awareness month. The statistic that has stayed with me since she has been diagnosed is that one child out of every five that are diagnosed dies. That's very powerful, and every September that passes, I am grateful that Paris is with me to see October and the following months to come.

At the beginning of October, Paris and I went to New York for her three-month follow-up scans. Unlike our last two follow-ups, this visit presented some new information, and it took me some time to gather my thoughts. The MRI of the spine was stable. The area by T10 remained unchanged. The MIBG was negative, all of which were good. The brain MRI, however, revealed an enhancement in the parietal lobe (right side of the brain) with a large adjacent vein having either a large thrombosis (blood clot) or leptomeningeal enhancement (swelling of the layer of tissue lining within the brain). This finding was not present on any of the previous scans.

The neurosurgeon and oncology team believed that the area was enhanced from an enlarged clotted blood vessel. However, since Paris has had neuroblastoma in the brain, they could not rule out the possibility of early neuroblastoma. Normal, everyday healthy people may experience a small thrombosis without even knowing it, and it would never cause a problem. But in Paris' case, any area that shows enhancement is reason for concern.

The team speculated that the enhancement may have been caused by infection (which is highly unlikely), an inflamed blood vessel that developed a blood clot from the chemo and radiation therapy that she endured over time, or possible neuroblastoma cells present within the tissue lining causing the area to swell. Some factors that put me more at ease were that Paris' urine markers were fine and there was no uptake or light up on the MIBG scan to detect disease. (However, the area could be so small that it wasn't picked up.) Plus the oncology team felt comfortable sending us home for two months. If they thought that it was neuroblastoma, they would have kept us in New York, and we would have devised a plan and begun treatment. When I asked them on a scale of 1 to 10 how worried they were about this area, they responded 1. When I weighed my pros and cons regarding the area, it led to a clotted blood vessel. To be safe, the team wanted to re-scan with a more advanced MRI of the brain in two months.

My initial reaction was if the area of uptake was really neuroblastoma I didn't want to wait two months to scan, for fear that the area would spread at a rapid rate, as neuroblastoma is an aggressive cancer and at that time clinical treatment for brain relapse was limited. We had already completed five cycles of oral chemo, and we had one main dose left of antibody 8H9. On the other hand, if we were to repeat the MRI scan too early, there most likely wouldn't be any change. So many decisions and so many possibilities with no concrete answers. After consultations, you just need to use your best judgment and follow your intuition. I opted for a happy medium. I would fly out with Paris in six weeks to repeat the MRI brain scan on more advanced machinery. If that area remained stable, we would fly back out to New York in January for her next three-month workup, which would include an MRI of the spine, MIBG injection/scan, CT scan, urine and bone marrows.

If you ever want to have an eye-opening experience, have a conversation with a 5-year-old cancer patient. While I was in clinic with Paris, we saw a family that we hadn't seen in a while. We got reacquainted and learned that the girl had relapsed and was undergoing treatment for the third time. All the kids are drawn to Paris because she's so young, and she ended up eating lunch with us as she waited for her treatment to begin. She spoke so diligently about her treatment plan, not sugar coating a single word. I was amazed that this 5-year-old girl could articulate everything without a doubt and be very matter of fact about it.

She began talking about Paris' hair. At the time, Paris had light brown, curly hair, which was her third hair after growing back differently after every round of chemo. This little girl was hairless and began to discuss her past hair types, which had also come back different every time. As she spoke, she was so confident despite her hardship. She stared at me with her bright blue crystal eyes and looked me dead in my eyes. There was a long pause, and then all of a sudden she asked me if my hair had always been straight.

I replied, "Yes."

She then said, "When my hair comes back, I wish it would come back just like yours: blonde and straight."

Let me tell you how hard it was for me to hold back the tears and answer, "I'm sure it will honey." A few days later, I learned that she unexpectedly passed. I'm confident she has the perfect hair type and color in heaven.

I had a few days to spare, as our scheduled flight was delayed. On that trip, I noticed that Paris would study the other children who didn't have hair. She looked as if she thought something looked different about them, but she couldn't put her finger on it. At one point, I thought she had noticed the difference, and since she is a very verbal child, I thought that she would ask directly why the other kids didn't have hair. I pondered what I would say to her, trying to think fast before she would ask. She just looked at them, glanced at me, stroked her own hair, and then continued playing. I continued to think about this scenario as the day progressed. I decided that when she asked, I would acknowledge her question by saying that everyone's hair grows differently and tell her that everyone may not look alike, but everyone is special in their own way.

Chapter 27: Paris and the School System

Children who have an area of concern in regard to cognitive, social/emotional, adaptive self-help skills, physical, occupational, or speech components are eligible for an evaluation from the school district in which they live by their 3rd birthday. School districts are obligated via Child Find to hold screenings. They look at health, vision/hearing, functional, academic, motor, communication, and social/emotional.

Paris was a candidate for the early intervention program, servicing children age 0-3 prior to entering the school district due to significant delays in gross motor skills. Although services could have been provided within my home directly from the state, we chose private therapy as it fit better into our schedule because we were traveling between different states and were hospitalized at great length over the course of two years. Since Paris had significant physical mobility needs due to the neuroblastoma and had been receiving private therapy since she was 9 months old, she was considered eligible to be evaluated through the school district upon turning 3 years old.

The purpose of the evaluation was to determine if she would qualify for special services within the school environment through an Individual Education Plan (IEP). The special education team, which consisted of the school nurse, school social worker, physical therapist, occupational therapist, speech and language therapist, and school psychologist, evaluated Paris in a play-based format. The team then gathered data, gave formal and informal screenings, some of which were researched based and others that were not, and determined if Paris would benefit from services that would assist her within either a self-contained or mainstreamed classroom environment for preschool.

On November 10, 2010, we had our IEP meeting to discuss the results of the evaluation, and I wondered if my sole was destined to do this job – both my career choice as a special education teacher and my role as a mother with a child who has cancer. I wondered if it was planned for me and that occurrences within my life were actually preparing me to do this. I analyzed various situations that I encountered and examined how and if they would prepare me to battle this, making me stronger along the way.

The meeting was very surreal for me based upon so many different factors, primarily because I have a degree in special education, and here I was sitting on the other side of the table as Paris received her IEP. Who better to advocate for my child than myself? This was another example of why I believe that things happen for a reason and your path takes you exactly where you should be in life.

When I was 17 years old, I worked retail, as probably many teenagers do after school or on weekends. At the time I just viewed it as a part time job, as a stepping stone to my work ethic and for experience purposes. I moved to Naperville in the summer of 2003 and quickly got hired as a special education teacher in the Naperville school district and then wanted to use my early childhood special education degree, so I applied for summer school. I worked the summer school program for three years and made many friends within the building. As I took Paris to the evaluation, I saw many familiar faces who remembered me from when I worked there. The school psychologist who assessed Paris was even a girl I used to work with at my retail job. It was so strange to cross paths again later in life. So I question, was I supposed to work within the district's preschool setting, and unbeknownst to me, be back there years later with my daughter?

Paris' cognitive functioning skills focused on reasoning, remembering, thinking, and problem solving. Her early academic and play skills were assessed using the Weschsler Preschool and Primary Scale of Intelligence, third edition. She scored superior, placing her within the 94 percentile. Paris' fine and gross motor skills were assessed using the Peabody Developmental Motor Scales-2. A motor quotient below 80 indicates a significant motor delay. Paris' overall gross motor quotient was 79, indicating a significant motor delay.

Paris qualified for special education services based on the results of the assessment under the category of other health impairment. She receives support services in the areas of physical therapy and adapted physical education and has access to a classroom instructional aide to accommodate her gross and fine motor needs within the classroom environment.

Special education accommodations are important to monitor through contact with your child's case manager, teacher, and principal. Inquire if the classroom teacher has noticed anything unusual with school performance. Make sure that you ask questions when things are unclear, document the conversations, keep paperwork in organized folders, and obtain copies of the data analysis and reports from teachers. Maintain a good relationship with the team of people, because they will be providing services to your child. The new model can qualify children under the Response to Intervention (RTI) model that will replace discrepancy in 2014. Children with a medical diagnosis may also be considered for a 504 plan, which will allow for certain accommodations within the classroom environment. New guidelines for 504 plans became broader in 2009, increasing accountability. By providing a 504 rather than an emergency medical plan, children have access to a special education teacher as their case manager. Emergency plans can be transferred into 504 plans if it is determined that learning challenges are a result of a medical diagnosis or treatment.

Chapter 28: Paris Goes to Preschool

I was giving Paris a bath a few days before her 3rd birthday and her follow-up scans, and I realized as I washed her long curly hair that these next couple of days may be the last time I am able to wash it and play with it using the soap suds or untangle it as the days get closer to returning to New York for her follow-up scans. I stared at the strands of hair that just naturally come out as I washed it. I carefully placed each strand on the side of the tub, looking at it. Most people don't ever have to wonder about having their children lose all of their hair when they take a bath. I do.

I have come to terms with the fact that every time her scans came around, I change as a person. I became moody and argumentative. I tended to bite all my hangnails off; my face would break out, my immune systems tended to suffer. I didn't eat properly. I felt sick. My lymph nodes would swell. This scan time, I felt even more anxious and noticed a change in my demeanor. Any time your child undergoes scans, you become nervous. The longer the scans are spread out and the more intense the treatment is, you begin to develop what they call "scanitisis" or "scanziety."

Paris' birthday in 2010 was a bittersweet day for me. Ralph and I kept saying how hard it was getting as Paris was getting older and becoming more conscious of what was happening to her during treatment and follow-up appointments. We remembered when we learned of the diagnosis that they hoped she would make it to 2 years old. We just kept saying we were going to try anything just to get her to 2. If we made it to 2, we would be lucky. Now she was 3 years old, and we had a clearer picture of this cancer and were more knowledgeable about the nature of neuroblastoma.

I was so grateful that Paris turned 3 years old and that she was alive to enjoy her birthday. Every birthday I had been told that her chances of survival were slim, and yet every year, she was here to celebrate her life with us. It was truly a miracle. I was torn by the fact that the very next day had the potential to send us right back into the treatment world again. The feeling could be compared to a person on parole. You enjoy the freedom that is given, but you can never really escape the reality of it. You're always one step away from being sent back to prison.

On a happier note, Bear Necessities offered to pay for Paris' 3rd birthday party, which I was very grateful for. There are good people out there in this world; I guess you just tend to notice them more clearly when bad things are happening around you. Last year at Paris' birthday, the owner of the pizza shop that contracts with the facility heard of her story and immediately felt a connection with her. He was a childhood cancer survivor and donated the pizzas to her party. Since we are having the same type of party again this year, I decided to contact the manager of the pizza shop again. I learned that he had decided to leave the pizza shop and go back to school, but the woman who had moved into his position was extremely interested in Paris' story. By the end of our conversation, she wanted to do the same thing for us and decided to donate pizzas as well. That night as I read Paris her bedtime stories, I told her to always remember to help people. You never know what type of impact you will have on someone. We had a wonderful day celebrating that Paris had turned 3 years old.

On her other birthdays, and really during her life, I never had the chance to reflect on being pregnant since I had been so focused and consumed with Paris' needs. For her third birthday, I was actually able to enjoy the day and not worry about medical concerns. I was able to focus on the story of how we brought Paris into the world and reminisce about the joy of having my baby. It was a perfect day.

After the party, we took Paris to the photo studio to take her third birthday pictures. I dressed her in a cute outfit where she wore tights and UGG boots. Paris walked with great difficulty due to the significant curvature in her spine, and it was obvious that her balance was off. She took big strides and swung her arms for balance. As we were awaiting our pictures, an older woman noticed Paris' pattern of walking. She decided it was her duty to stop my sister and say, "You know, I think she's having a hard time walking in those UGG boots, don't you think?"

I just want to say to everyone reading this book, please keep your comments to yourself because you really don't have any idea what you're talking about when you approach people, and you end up sounding like an ass. Trust me, I will politely call you on the fact that you're sounding like an idiot and disregard your intruding comment. Please don't feel the need to comment on parenting, on appearance, on what the kid is eating at whatever time of day, on if they didn't finish their food first before a dessert, on what they're wearing regardless of the weather, on if they talk bossy in public, on if they throw a tantrum in public, or on if you think they are too old to ride in a stroller or have a pacifier, a bottle, or a favorite toy/blanket. Unless you witness a parent beating their child in broad daylight, I recommend you just keep your comments to yourself. My sister turned to her before I could even respond and bluntly stated, "It's not the shoes. She has cancer, which affects the way she walks."

The very next day after Paris' birthday, we headed to New York for her brain MRI to reassess the new enhancement. When we got on the plane, I continued my roller coaster of emotions. It was truly a high/low dynamic. I had felt overjoyed that Paris was able to enjoy every aspect of her birthday, as every child should, without having to worry about anything medically related. However, today I am faced with getting on the plane and putting her through another IV stick to undergo a scan that may change our lives again. It was sad to me because Paris also went from being so happy and excited about her birthday to worrying about why we were headed back to New York.

Thanksgiving fell on November 23, 2010, and that year I could say that we had been truly blessed with good health. It is a small thing that is often taken for granted. Paris' brain MRI showed that the area in question was still present; however it had not changed and resembled more of a vessel rather than disease. Needless to say, this would be another area that the team would be watching very closely on future scans. We would still go back in January for her scheduled three-month scans – this one was just an added bonus. That meant we would be home for the holidays again. Paris would also start preschool on November 29, and she was all ready for it.

Those scan results led us to have to make some good, complicated normal decisions. If we wanted Paris to begin preschool after Thanksgiving break, we would have to place her with a new daycare provider, Mrs. Diane, who lived within our school district's boundary lines, so Paris would receive transportation to and from preschool. This would mean a lot of new changes for Paris within a week's time. We thought that Paris only lives once, and we live within our case's three-month intervals, so we decided to give Paris the opportunity to experience school.

On November 29, 2007, exactly three years before her first day of preschool, Paris was diagnosed with neuroblastoma. That was the date that the doctors gave us some of the worst news that a parent could hear, and I vividly remember thinking I would not have the opportunity to see her experience milestones such as going to school. Today she attended preschool with her peers, and both Ralph and I were there to see her experience it. To the average parent, having their child attend preschool at 3 years old or kindergarten at 5 years old may be considered a routine thing to do, but to us, to parents with a child who has cancer, it meant so much more than just an act, it was an accomplishment symbolizing that Paris had endured so much just to be fortunate enough to experience what the average child experiences.

That moment to see Paris walk through the preschool classroom door and quickly adjust to the routine made me so happy. She fit right into the class, and as I waved goodbye, she gave me the look that meant that she was going to be fine and to please stop embarrassing her with the waving and the well wishes. She has been used to going with so many people that it didn't bother her that some strange woman picked her up and walked away with her. After thinking about it, I would rather have a child that adjusts well and I be the one nervous all day rather than have a crying child who is unable to adjust to the classroom environment. She enjoyed preschool so much. She enjoyed the routine and looked forward to working with her teachers and seeing her friends at school.

Chapter 29: Contemplating a Second Baby and ALK

In December 2010, the infamous topic of having another child when you have one that is sick was seriously debated. Everyone seemed to have an opinion on it. People either were in favor of the idea of expanding your family or they were against it, but ultimately it's your decision to choose to have another baby. With everything comes difficulty, and there will be much more sacrifice needed with two children – one child with cancer and the other without – but I thought to myself, after all that I have been through thus far, can it really get worse?

In the general public view, this is a great debate, and the truth is that many people who have a child diagnosed with cancer decide to have more children and some families decide to have just one. Families that learn of their child's diagnosis of neuroblastoma battle with many factors to consider, such as their personal age and energy level, their child's age of diagnosis, finances, work strains, and relationship foundations. As I accompanied Paris to her intensive treatments, the hospital is always required to ask, "Is there a chance you could be pregnant?"

I just wanted to laugh out loud, thinking okay, I'm in another state, away from my husband, dealing with all of this stress, not in the mood, I feel like a mess, and I'm tired all of the time. I seriously don't think that I'm pregnant. But I would always politely say no. I would think about the possibility of another child all the time but was conflicted because Paris needed us both, and with another child and one in treatment, someone would always have to be away. We agreed that if God permitted, Paris would have the opportunity to be a big sister. Time would only tell. I believed that having another baby would be a blessing in itself.

There was also great debate on the reasons to have another baby once you have a child with cancer. The blood cord of another child can be crucial and may be used to aide in treatment plans. Viacord has a program called Sibling Connection that pays for the initial processing fee of $2,195 and a five-year storage fee of $125 if you already have a child with a qualifying illness. If a sibling matches the criteria and they are full siblings, then you qualify for the program.

In my opinion, if another child allows Paris the opportunity to be healed from neuroblastoma by using blood cord material, then that is an additional blessing. How wonderful would it be for a sibling to know that they gave life to their brother or sister at a time when he or she needed it most? In my opinion, it should not be looked at as wrong or as the other child produced to cure the other or as a replacement child, but simply as an addition that can possibly save the life of a sibling and bring joy to the family.

Ralph and I had some real conversations regarding the future of our relationship and the reality of Paris' disease. At this point of my life, I could talk with people about Paris and her cancer and speak very frankly, separating fact from emotion. People would be in awe when I could say without breaking down that "Paris has a less than 5 percent survival rate due to the number of relapses and specific areas that the tumor has affected, and being that she has questionable spots that remain, every time that there is a relapse, it decreases her chances of overall survival." I guess people were shocked that her chances were poor medically speaking since she looked so good on the outside.

Ralph and I were very aware that Paris was a true blessing, and her survival thus far was nothing but a miracle from a medical standpoint. She should have passed on at day 10, age 1, or surely by age 2. Now Paris was 3 years old, but there was always a risk of relapse and that our worst fears would come true. After Paris initially became sick, Ralph and I made a rather quick decision for him to get a vasectomy to avoid this from ever happening to us again. Well, three years later we decided that may not have been the best choice. Despite all of the hardships we have endured, Paris has brought so much joy to us as parents that we couldn't fathom the idea of not having her around or the reality of us never being able to be parents in the event that something happened to her. During the summer, Ralph consulted with various vasectomy reversal specialists within Illinois, but he ultimately went to Arizona to get it reversed by Dr. Marks. Everyone that I spoke to about this had the exact same comment, "Ralph must love you a lot to consciously know what it feels like and then to go back and do it again."

Here is the letter that I wrote to thank Dr. Marks and his team:

Dear Dr. Marks and the ICVR team,
After months of searching and consulting for a vasectomy reversal doctor within Illinois and having been told that our chances of success were poor, we decided to expand our search, and we came across the ICVR team. We researched your site, read your bio, and immediately were impressed. After speaking to you that night during our consultation, it confirmed that we had met a very unique and genuine individual who we would choose to give Ralph the opportunity to become fertile and possibly conceive again.

During that two-hour consultation, you became a part of our family. As you listened to our story regarding Paris' health, you confirmed that the decision that we made to have the initial vasectomy was simply a decision that was made at the time of chaos; not good or bad. You gave us success rates, and we genuinely felt a connection with you after learning that you switched professions from dealing with cancer to providing people the chance to be truly happy.

I greatly appreciated the regular updates from your team during the surgery. It gave me comfort knowing what was happening while I wasn't there. With every person you meet, you have the opportunity to learn something from them. I'm glad that Ralph's challenge provided you with new information. I was very excited to learn that despite the difficulties presented, Ralph's success rate was 90 to 97 percent.

The power of being a parent is a very special gift, and to have a child with an unfortunate disease that can potentially take her away makes you realize just how special being a parent can be and makes you realize just how much you can love another unconditionally. We are extremely grateful that you were able to perform the vasectomy reversal and provide us with the opportunity to expand our family, providing Paris with either a brother or sister.

It was difficult to be told by others that the chances of success were not high and that they wished that they could do more considering our situation. Then somehow, at just the right time, we came across you and your team with the mission to make men dads again. We value your experience to be able to not just do one universal "one size fits all" procedure, but to instead carefully analyze the precise type of procedure to be used per patient by examining each one carefully to decide which procedure is best to implement for best success rates.

You are a very special person with a great purpose in life. The team you work with is extraordinary. Ralph and I believe that through this entire ordeal over the past two years that it is very clear as day that you're destined to meet certain people at just the right time in your life when you least expect it and need it most. We will be in touch very soon, and then you will be able to add Baby Strickland to your baby photo wall.

During Paris' January 2011 appointment, I inquired about ALK genetic testing for children with neuroblastoma. Neuroblastoma can be inherited if the germline mutations in the anaplastic lymphoma kinase (ALK gene) are present, causing hereditary neuroblastoma.

The genetic team at Sloan-Kettering decided to test a piece of a tumor sample that they had frozen from one of her past surgeries. If the sample came back negative, then Paris had an isolated random case without an explanation. If the sample came back positive, then Ralph and I would need to send out our own blood samples to determine if there is a familial gene. The team warned that the cost of this type of procedure is often not covered under insurance plans and is costly. I called the hospital's financial aid department, and they told me I was still covered under the financial agreement until February 24, 2011. That meant the testing would be covered under the hospital in its entirety or the remainder left over, after what had been submitted to my insurance company, would not be charged and would be our responsibility.

I became more interested and concerned if in fact Paris was a case of "bad luck" or if she indeed had the genetic mutation for neuroblastoma, meaning that Ralph or I would be a carrier unbeknownst to us. Neuroblastoma is so random. There are cases that have no ALK gene link, which make it a fluke as to why the child was exposed, and then there are some that indicate gene mutations; however the mutations among children can vary. We went ahead with the testing and would find out the results in February.

Chapter 30: Preparing for Spine Surgery

It was really a blessing to be at home for the holidays with an uneventful status. Looking back, I realized that we had spent all of the holidays thus far in the hospital. Our first Christmas was obviously not the perfect situation for me. I had pictured being at home with a huge Christmas tree with decorations, presents all around, holiday music, huge dinners, and family, but it was just the opposite. I found myself instead surrounded by a roommate at the hospital. Volunteers at the hospital provided bags full of gifts for children. People of many different ethnicities dressed as Santa and came to greet all the children, even if that meant entering the room in a yellow gown covering their festive attire. I felt such gratitude to receive this memory but wished it was different. Paris didn't know the difference, so we tried to make the best of it. When you have the chance, help families around Christmas or donate items to hospitals to kids who aren't able to be in the comfort of their own home during the holidays because through the good nature of others is how we created our memories.

Our appointment for our routine three-month scan work-up in New York was scheduled for January 4th through January 7th. We flew using Corporate Angels Network, which provides families free travel on private company jets that fly on routine business to access the best medical treatment across the country at no cost. Paris underwent an MRI of the brain/spine, MIBG injection and scan, and bone marrows. The results of the scan were stable – no new disease and the new spot on the frontal lobe was still present but unchanged, therefore they were still attributing it to being a blood vessel. The team would continue to monitor Paris every three months in New York, so our next scans would be sometime in April. Paris continued to be on no treatment plan at that time. The team tested her PHA levels to see if she could receive some of the vaccinations that she was never able to receive since she began treatment at 10 days old.

Because the scans had been stable, it was time to go ahead and plan for the corrective spine surgery, which would place growing rods in attempt to improve the 56 degree curvature. We would do the surgery in Chicago because both the specialists in Chicago and in New York collaborated and agreed on the same plan. Doing the surgery in Chicago would allow me to be closer to home, still work, and have family support. We had a consultation with the orthopedic surgeon scheduled for Monday, January 10, to finalize our surgery date, which would give Paris just enough time to recover and then jump right back into scan schedules.

I had contacted Dr. Kramer to request that since Paris was having scans every three months, perhaps the bone marrow test could be alternated every other visit, as we had never had bone marrow involvement. I later received an email requesting that I call her at my earliest convenience. I immediately called her back, and she informed me that she would prefer to continue to conduct bone marrow aspirations every three months because they were an indicator to determine potential secondary cancers that may occur over time due to all of the chemotherapy.

She also told us that she found partial trical #1. The "normal healthy" person has 46 chromosomes. But Paris' bone marrow tests in July revealed an additional chromosome. This would need to be further monitored by a fluorescence in situ hybridization (FISH) test used to detect the presence or absence of a specific DNA sequence on chromosomes. Paris' secondary risk cancer is leukemia, which is a cancer of blood cells. When one is diagnosed with leukemia, the body produces large numbers of abnormal or immature blood cells. Since blood cells originate in the bone marrow, the most common places to detect leukemia are either through blood tests or by conducting a bone marrow aspirate and biopsy. Dr. Kramer stated that a deleted number 5, 7, or 8 chromosome typically indicates oncoming leukemia. These chromosomes were not missing in Paris' case when the bone marrow biopsy was reviewed; therefore her scans were not indicating oncoming leukemia at this time. However, the team must monitor the additional chromosome through the use of a FISH test at least twice a year.

I scheduled Paris' spine surgery. It was a necessary measure, and being that we had a healthy stretch and three-month intervals to work with, Ralph and I decided to schedule it for March 15, 2011.
I met with various specialists regarding Paris' spine, and the specialists in both Chicago and New York recommend the placement of growth/growing rods. Growing rods are not permanent and allow the bones to grow and expand in addition to aiding in straightening out her spine by at least 20 degrees. Her curve was very significant, at 56 degrees. Curves to her degree are usually seen in older patients. Placing the growing rods would not fix the problem; however it would significantly improve it, to about 36 degrees. These metal rods would be placed and surgically adjusted every six months. The structures usually last for two years and then need to be replaced. The surgery would be between four and six hours, and she would have approximately five days recovering in the hospital and another three weeks to fully recover.

She was very active, so the main risk was that the rods tend to break over time, meaning that an entire new structure would have to be surgically implanted. However, if we did not do the surgery, her back would permanently curve and fuse, which would cause a severe deformity. The curve over time would continue to press against her lung, which down the line would cause breathing problems because she would not be able to expand her lungs to full capacity.

Chapter 31: New Challenges Await

On February 4, I received an email from Dr. Kramer's office with the results from the genetic test for the potential ALK gene. They came back negative. Paris' tumor sample did not contain the ALK gene, which means that her tumor was the result of a fluke upon conception rather than Ralph or myself carrying the specific gene, causing a mutation. Typically children who are diagnosed at such a young age have the ALK gene present. Again, this is somewhat atypical for Paris' case. This again confirmed that all neuroblastoma cases vary and she again beat the odds of what is expected.

Later that month, Paris would have her PHA levels tested so she could begin the re-immunization process. She received her vaccination schedule and was eligible to receive her vaccines at 3 years old – 1 year and 5 months after the completion of chemotherapy.

On March 11, 2011, Sendai, Japan, was struck by a devastating 9.0 megathrust earthquake that lasted six minutes and triggered a 23-foot tsunami, which caused mass destruction. The natural disaster eventually caused radioactivity from the Fukushima nuclear power plant to leak into the air, and Japan declared a nuclear emergency. Hearing the news of mass panic of people trying to avoid high levels of radiation seemed surreal to me. As I watched the news and saw people dressed in protective gear and witnessed people being scanned with the Geiger counter to detect levels of incurred radiation, I quickly reverted to the thought that Paris and other children who obtain MIBG scans and are purposefully injected with levels of radiation to identify areas of potential cancer. They are radioactive for weeks after injection. So people in Japan were obviously trying to avoid levels of radiation, and I sit with Paris every three months for the doctors to purposefully inject her with radiation.

The news reported having iodine readily available to reverse the effect of radiation exposure, and I couldn't help but think to myself that I had an abundance of iodine (SSKI drops) on hand, as I had to give Paris the seven drops the day before, the day of, and the day after the MIBG scan.

We had Paris' final consultation with the orthopedic surgeon the evening of March 11 and discussed the procedures regarding her upcoming surgery. The surgery was scheduled for March 15 in Chicago. She would have growing rods placed, allowing the spine to be expanded every 6 months rather than fused together with a permanent rod. She would also have titanium rods placed, most likely along the muscle, with the screws attached to the ribs, which would go downward and connect to the pelvic area, packing some bone-to-bone graph to fuse the screws so they would be more solid. However, since she was so small, the surgeon would have to decide exactly which method of connection works well during the surgery. He seemed to still be unsure of how he wanted to anchor the rods and was trying to decide which way would be best for her.

She was expected to have to wear a full-time thoraco lumbo sacral orthosis (TLSO) brace. He said that she would be sore, swollen, and on pain medication, but that kids her age are very resilient. He expected her to be out of school for approximately four weeks after surgery. However, that number is a generic time frame and would be determined more specifically after the surgery, when he would advise on specific physical therapy needs.

The structure itself would be able to be felt and mildly seen underneath the skin. One concern was that the actual device may break or crack over time. He compared it to a paperclip wiggling, due to her being a normal active young child. If you bend it so much, it becomes flimsy and can weaken, which then would mean it would need to be replaced. He told us we may not even know if the structure is cracked or weakened, but she would complain more of back pain or it would become visible on an x-ray. This was why he wanted her to wear the TLSO for additional support and to solder the area toward the bottom of the spine with additional bone graphing material to better hold the screws and rods in place.

Paris had her spinal surgery on March 15, 2011, at Children's Memorial Hospital. We arrived at 6 a.m., and I took her back at 8:20 a.m. She fell asleep quickly by the cherry-flavored gas that filled her little mask. I walked away, questioning and debating, "Am I or am I not doing the right thing?" I just kept telling myself all the factors that favor doing it now and that every specialist had recommend it to avoid a more significant curve and ultimately to avoid a permanent deformity.

The thought of surgery near the spine just overwhelmed my mind. What if something goes wrong and the decision I made to help her actually risks her ability to move and causes her not to be able to walk? The thought of being just one nerve away from making a mistake, the thought of this as the first surgery not to remove a tumor, the thought that I actually had time to plan this surgery rather than be told that they found a tumor and tomorrow we would have surgery to remove it, leaving me no time to process it but just react. So, I left her with a million thoughts racing in my mind, as I walked two feet down the hallway. I reached the waiting room and met my family who surrounded Ralph and me. The four to six hour wait began. Tick tock…tick tock…have you ever noticed that time moves so slow when you're waiting for something?

I received many calls that day from friends, family, other parents that we know whose children also have neuroblastoma, as well as parents whose children passed but still show so much emotional and verbal support despite how hard it is for them. I got one call in particular that was very special. While in New York, we met a family whose daughter had neuroblastoma. Ralph had become close friends with her dad, Mark, during his stays in New York, as there are not many dads at the Ronald McDonald House. Mark shared that he had gotten into an accident as an adult and needed a permanent rod to correct his spine, so he could relate to Paris' next step. He was always in awe when he learned of Paris' trials and tribulations at such a young age. He was always concerned and genuinely cared about her. When he learned that we were in the process of scheduling the surgery, he called and left messages offering to be there to talk, as he had gone through the surgery himself. Unfortunately, shortly after he made the phone call to us, he unexpectedly passed away. The day of Paris' surgery, his wife sent me a message that said, "Just wanted to let you guys know that we will be thinking about you today as Paris goes through surgery. We know all will go well, as Mark will watch over her. He will be there holding her hand. He loved her and you guys. I told him this morning that I know he is always here with Megan and I, but today Paris, you, and Ralph need him, so go be with Paris and keep her safe."

The friends we have made along this journey are indescribable. They became our family – it's that simple. I believe with all my heart and felt that Mark was one of the angels in that room with Paris for 10 hours, comforting her and keeping her safe throughout the procedure. I received the first call at 10:20 a.m. that they made the first incision and that the spine was exposed. The calls are similar to what I would expect a secret service call to be like – you're on the phone for less than a minute and given a brief update and a confirmation that they will call you back. At 1:04 p.m. I received the second call that said they were placing the hardware (screws and plates), and at 3:08 p.m. I got the third call that they were placing the rods and that it would be another two hours to complete.

That caller stated that her nerve monitoring throughout the process did not indicate anything unusual during surgery. The surgeon called us at 5:15 p.m. and said that she was recovering in ICU and that the surgery went well with no complications. He noticed an immediate improvement of approximately 20 to 30 degrees, which was unexpected (I think he was surprised himself), as he had said during our consultation not to expect to notice any changes right away, that it would be a slow progress and only slightly noticeable every six months when they adjusted the rods. Needless to say it was a long 10 hours. He changed his placement ideas once he had her spine exposed. He decided to shave off some of her own unneeded vertebrae to use as bone graphing material in addition to artificial bone to solder the rods to ensure a secure placement. This added to the surgery time.

Ralph and I met her in the ICU, and to our surprise she looked good. She was not as swollen as we had anticipated compared to other surgeries. She was moving her legs and toes and was receiving morphine every 10 minutes, watching Disney movies, eating popsicles, and resting. She commented that "her back has an ouchie," but then went back to sleep as she pushed the pain button. My whole family rotated shifts to stay with her during the day and overnight at the hospital. One night when it was my turn, I looked at her and had an image flash before me. I once read that 67 percent of mothers suffer from post-traumatic stress. In that moment, I completely envisioned her bald again, and my mind immediately reverted back to her in treatment. I had to reach over and move her hair to almost snap me out of it.

The team scheduled an x-ray for the following day to determine exactly how much of an improvement there was. Paris would be inpatient for another four to five days and have to wear the TLSO brace all day when at home for stability and protection. The team would assess her, and I was sure I'd get a list of restrictions. She would then have the rods adjusted every six months to expand her spine to hopefully an even straighter degree.

Paris used the next day to rest, and I used it to familiarize myself with all of the new restrictions that came with the healing process. Where do I even begin? There was so much to remember and to be cautious of.

- No twisting or trunk rotation. Paris must log roll for all rolling and when turning while standing, she must keep shoulders in line with her pelvis.
- No lifting shoulders above 90 degrees.
- No bending hips greater than 90 degrees.
- No lying on her stomach.
- Must wear a TLSO brace at all times.
- Perform strengthening activities two to three times per day that focus on tightening the buttock muscles and strengthening the quadriceps.

The luck was on our side on St. Patrick's Day, as it was the first day that Paris got out of bed and walked with a great amount of assistance from the hospital bed to the hospital room door. She needed an x-ray to determine exactly how much her spine had improved since surgery. Ralph and I brought her down to the x-ray area at Children's Memorial Hospital and had to maneuver her from the wheelchair to the long table to remove the brace and then somehow carry her to this hard wooden chair devise without the brace to obtain an upright x-ray. Mind you, this was one day out of surgery and the first time she was out of bed and had to be moved without the sacred brace on, and neither Ralph nor I had any "training" on how to really move her. Who wants to guess how much swearing, debating, and arguing was done that day in front of the x-ray tech as we attempted this stressful situation on our own? Eventually we were able to complete the task and get the x-ray done. The x-ray tech probably had her own opinion of us, and it gave us another opportunity to examine how we work as a team in stressful situations. We were able to catch a glimpse of the newly structured spine x-ray, and it was gorgeous. It was so much straighter, I couldn't believe it. Looking at the remarkable image made me believe that all of that questioning back and forth on whether or not to do the surgery was answered immediately – it was clear as day.

Paris was discharged from the hospital the evening of Monday, March 21. By Tuesday morning, she was no longer attached to any medical devices, all the IVs were out and she was back at home. Paris thought that meant that she was all better and could resume her daily activities, picking up where she left off. In reality, it meant Paris had to be given specific rules about what she could and could not do at home. She could no longer reach for things that were above her head. She could not twist, jump, turn, bend down, roll, do her leg lift trick, climb the stairs, get in and out of bed on her own, sit upright, use the potty, take a bath, or basically do anything independently for approximately four weeks, until after our post-operative follow-up appointment.

We explained to her that she just had surgery on her back and her back had an ouchie. We told her it needed time to heal, so until it healed, there were things she couldn't do. We added that when it healed, she would be able to do everything like before. We made sure that she understood that she needed to ask for help with everything and ask before she did anything. These were challenges within themselves.

Paris became frustrated with some of the new restrictions. For example, prior to the surgery, we were trying to potty train Paris and asked her to tell us when she felt like she had to go to the bathroom. We told her that we didn't want her to go in the diaper and that she needed to sit on the potty when she felt like she had to use the bathroom. After her surgery, however, when Paris would say that she had to use the potty, we would respond, "Paris you are going to have to go in your diaper since you can't sit on the potty right now."

She would say, "But I can't. I have to sit on the potty or I won't get my potty treat," and begin to cry. It was just a confusing message for her.

Everything was turned upside down for her. She wanted to continue to try to do things all by herself and started to push us away saying,

"I'm a big girl. I can do it all by myself...let me show you." I have to admire her determined personality, but at the same time, it broke my heart because she simply didn't fully understand. So many new challenges awaited her. She was now given a "new spine," so she needed to adapt and learn how to balance and maneuver with a straighter spine rather than the 56-degree curve that she was used to. Straightening the spine made her taller by a few inches, and she didn't have a lot of strength in her legs and lower torso. She basically did not know how to work those muscles, as she has never had to use them. She was told to wear the TLSO brace all day for support as the spine healed and to limit her habit of naturally reverting to curving to the right. She had to re-learn how to walk at 3 years old.

As I watched her, I would think to myself thank God this surgery was without any complications. I was grateful that I was overcoming these challenges with her and that we had the opportunity to face them. I had to carry her as she transitioned from a laying down position to an upright position as we went up and down the stairs. I couldn't help but think to myself what if something had gone wrong during surgery and she became permanently immobile. How would I have explained to her when she asked when would she be able to run or walk again? I was very grateful that God guided this particular orthopedic surgeon that day and that there were no complications and that I am blessed not to have that conversation with her.

My mom watched Paris for the first week home after being discharged from the hospital and then every Thursday after. One day, she decided to play doctor and brought out her doctors kit. She began to role play her experience of taking pain medication orally after having been weaned from the morphine IV drip. She told my mom, "I'll be the nurse and you be the patient. Pretend you're sick. I'm gonna give you the bad medicine." She took out the syringe and pretended it was filled with medicine. She told my mom, "Okay it's time to take your bad medicine. Open your mouth." She instructed her to cry while yelling at her to take it as she squeezed her cheeks. In this situation, she took the dominant role and became the person giving the medicine rather than the person taking it. We had to discuss with her that sometimes when we are sick we have to take medicine that tastes bad to make us feel better, even if we don't like it, again another confusing message.

My spring break fell during Paris' second week of recovery, so I was able to be home with her. I also had to make the thousands of phone calls that come with the territory of surgery. I called the insurance company since we had extended our expected stay in the hospital, already dealing with the bills that were just accrued two weeks ago. I called the nurse case manager, Paris' daycare and school, and the team in New York. I made follow-up appointments, faxed Paris' restrictions to her school and private physical therapist, made upcoming physical therapist appointments, scheduled home-bound services with the school since she has been out for 10 consecutive school days, and scheduled a follow-up IEP meeting to inform them of her restrictions. In between all that, Paris took her first four independent steps toward me. Once she realized that she could accomplish that, she wanted to continue to display her newfound ability and continually said, "I can do it all by myself. Let me go!" I stayed close behind her to guide her every step. It was so wonderful to see her so proud of herself and to see that she was making great progress.

On April 3, I received the bill in the mail from Children's Memorial Hospital, which encompassed all of the services from Paris' recent surgery, including the private hospital room, intermediate care, surgery/operating costs, medication from the pharmacy, surgical supplies, prosthetics/orthotics, the implants/devices, blood products/transfusions, radiology, anesthesia, and physical therapy costs from March 15 to 21. The grand total was $121,456.12.

Chapter 32: The What Ifs

A woman named Norma Reardon coined the term "scanxiety-psychosis" and said it is characterized by "irritability, loss of sleep, crying uncontrollably, nausea, vomiting, heart palpitations, hyperventilating, headaches, loss of ability to think clearly, loss of ability to remember, loss of appetite, or inability to stop eating, pacing, sweating, staring blankly into space, facial tics, and nonsensical muttering. Subjects should be assumed armed and dangerous. Approach with extreme caution, especially if you are a doctor. Attempts at humor, perkiness, or inane platitudes are at your own risk."

Every time we approach our three-month scans, I typically feel very anxious, sad, nervous, and grumpy. I may subconsciously instigate fights with my family, stress myself out so much that I miss my menstrual cycle altogether, get headaches and stomach aches, throw up, don't eat, can't sleep, overwork to distract myself or feel overwhelmed by any little thing. I begin to think what if we get thrown right back into the routine of treatment after Paris has been exposed to a degree of calmness? Ralph reminds me, "Why be sad twice? Things are good now, so don't focus on the sad possibilities beforehand, otherwise you will miss out on this valuable time with Paris now. If and when it comes time to deal with sadness, then we will."

I found myself wondering about the "what if's," looking back at my past to determine how or why I got to certain stages of my life. What if's play a big role when you are faced with neuroblastoma. The fact is that there is a chance it could come back, regardless of whether you preventively treat it or not. It's really all a gamble. As a mother you know what your child can handle and what they can't. You tend to have an insight that only you know. Other people may not agree with you or understand your rationale, but I have found that you need to be comfortable with the decisions you make for your child and ultimately do what's right for them.

You can't step into that world of what if, because it only contains negativity. I have, however, at times surrounded myself with negative thoughts, which ultimately makes me sad at the realistic possibilities that no one should ever be faced with. It's hard to see the positive, and you feel stuck in a cycle of horrible thoughts. You can't live your life in the what if's. You have to live your life for the now. Those thoughts are meaningless. Why worry about what is going to happen in the future? It's not going to change the current situation. It's only going to change your current mood.

I sometimes find myself thinking about what it would be like to not have Paris with me. They are very strange thoughts, but they do cross my mind. I try to place myself in these situations because in reality, it could very well happen, as neuroblastoma is a vicious disease. There's really never any safe zone, just a continuous hope that it will never return. Maybe it is, because I hear too many stories of children passing away and I truly feel their pain. I almost want to somewhat mentally prepare myself for the absolute worst, even though I know you can never prepare yourself for that type of situation or loss. I ask myself, could I live in the same house that we all once did? Would her spirit know where to find me? Could I enter her room or ever change the décor? Could I give away her clothes or toys? Could I ever love another child like I love her or stand to look at her pictures without crying? Could I ever function through the days to come, overcome holidays or special events? Could I watch other children who may have resembled her? Sometimes I think thoughts have the potential to create insanity. Again, my rule is to allow the thoughts to enter but not consume me and to remember that it's pointless to think about things that don't exist. Remember to focus on the present because the fears you have for the future may never happen. There's a possibility that Paris may never encounter neuroblastoma again after this journey, and I'll have spent all of my time thinking about the what if's, allowing those thoughts to take over my happy moments now with her.

When you're a parent of a healthy child, you would never think about the death of your child. If you are a parent of a child with a chronic illness, however, you are constantly thinking about the what if's, and a lot of the time that involves the possibility of death. The thought of what if my child dies? What would I do? Would I be able to hold my marriage together knowing that the child that was made up of both of us is no longer present? Would we be able to cope and work through such a loss? Would I be able to attend the funeral? What would I say? Would I ever "get over it"? Would I ever be able to be around another baby? Would I ever be able to have another baby? Would I ever be who I was when I lost such a part of me?

In late April, Paris and Ralph flew to New York for Paris' three-month routine scans. The team at Memorial Sloan-Kettering has decided that Paris no longer needs CT scans. She still receives an MRI of the brain and spine, MIBG injection and scan, and bone marrow aspirations. Paris knows every time she boards the plane that she is headed to New York and anticipates getting an IV. On this trip, she told Ralph that she didn't like it and didn't want to get the IV anymore because she felt fine. We reminded her that she needed to continue to have checkups and that she needed to be brave.

I received Paris' results, and the MRI of the brain looked stable, noting the "stable curvilinear enhancing structure in the right parietal lobe without significant change." The impression states that there was "no evidence for new or progressive intracranial disease." The MRI of the spine continued to note a "stable enhancing nodule measuring 10 x 6 millimeters along the right T10 transverse process/proximal right 10th rib." The bone marrow results were also considered stable; however they indicated 1 percent of cells with an extra piece of chromosome 1.

Although Paris' prognosis was good, we had many close friends who relapsed or passed during April and May of 2011. It seemed that neuroblastoma had decided to strike the cancer world with a vengeance.

Our friend's daughter relapsed in December 2010, and they anticipated her having an additional 6 months to 1 year to live. Her mother became desperate and began to seek out systemic/holistic methods of treatments, as the hospitals had stated that the options were limited. I don't cast judgment on anyone trying to save their child. I know firsthand in that situation that if someone told me to do anything, even if it sounded ridiculous, I would in attempts to save my child. However, from a clear perspective as a parent, you also need to recognize when it's time to accept the things you cannot change and when to let them go, as hard as that is. Our friend decided to try a remedy using mud from bloodroot as a last attempt. Her child was covered in this solution in attempts to save her. Other parents have had their children drink proposed concoctions, perform rituals, and do basically anything anyone recommended in attempts to save their life. Parents will go great lengths in attempts to save their child, no matter the cost or no matter how silly it may seem. Whichever method suits you at the time is what's best for you. However, parents should remain cautious of individuals that prey on those who are desperate and seeking one last option, proposing remedies that are unrealistic.

***

Everyone has a defining moment in their lives, when they realize just what life is really about. Situations make us realize that we are human and that everything else before cancer was trivial. I found myself reflecting on the fact that I wouldn't have spent more than a few minutes or the length of the commercial feeling sorry for those who were going through this disease then. Ultimately, I'd go back into my routine of everyday life. Did I ever take action? Did I ever question what I could do to help those in need? Situations like the ones I have faced give me a strong sense of reality – life is about valuing every moment with the ones you love and not taking anything for granted. Sometimes it takes these situations that make us realize that life is teaching us a lesson about what is real and not real. Until you are faced with almost losing a child, then and only then does the concept of how valuable life really is sinks in.

My friend introduced me to her group of girlfriends, and as I was being introduced, I could see that they had already been informed of my situation beforehand. It was hard to watch their "healthy" children play, and it really hit home to me that I'm "that" mom. I'm the one who has to worry about days that "might" happen. I listened to them as they stated how grateful they are and how they needed to take a better look at their situation because they are blessed and not focus on the minor issues that arise on a daily basis. I felt the consensus that they were really saying, "I'm really glad I'm not in your situation." When I discussed my feelings with my husband, he presented his position on the issue. He's been the topic of similar conversations and feels grateful if he is the reason that other parents reflect on their children. That they ultimately become more involved, are less angry at the little things, and allow their children to be kids, let go of their tight grip and alleviate fears they have, ultimately understanding that life is not promised and today should be valued to its full potential.

I am so grateful when I do not have to constantly be at the hospital, taking blood samples, chemo, radiation, and antibodies, deciding which protocol to choose, watching my child engulfed with sadness and pain. I really do value the time without that aspect in my life even though I know it is always there, just put on hold for a bit. Scans can determine your fate and re-adjust your life in an instant.

Chapter 33: Catching Up on Vaccinations

In May, Paris' pediatrician gave us a road map to catch her up with her vaccine schedule. Her PHA levels were finally within a normal range; therefore she was eligible to receive them.

The rotavirus vaccine, which prevents against extreme diarrhea and dehydration, is typically given at 2, 4, and 6 months. Paris was unable to receive it at those times because of her cancer. She actually had been exposed to the virus while on treatment, and in turn suffered from extreme dehydration and diarrhea. At three years old, she was too old to receive the vaccine; therefore she was waived from that particular one.

The oncology team and her pediatrician urged her to have the diphtheria, tetanus, and pertussis (DtaP), inactivated poliovirus vaccine (IPV), haemophilus influenzae type b (HIB) to protect against meningitis, and pneumococcal conjugate (Prevnar) to protect against disease caused by the bacterium streptococcus pneumoniae. These four shots would be given every two months for three cycles. Once the doctor assessed the vaccine response from the primary series, Paris would then be given the hepatitis B vaccine, which consists of one shot for three cycles. Paris had received one dose of the hepatitis B vaccine at birth. The final single shot, which is the measles, mumps, and rubella vaccine (MMR), is typically given at 2 months, after completing the hepatitis series.

On June 3, Paris rode a tricycle and moved her legs to pedal the bike all by herself! It was amazing to see my 3 and a half year old accomplish this goal. She enjoyed making the tricycle go so fast and feel the wind go through her hair as she pedaled quickly. She quickly mastered steering the bike as she pedaled down the block and screamed, "This is so fun mommy!"

A week later, I received a call from Dr. Kramer, as I had asked her to contact me regarding Paris' recent scan results and questions I had regarding her bone marrow results. The first question Dr. Kramer always asked was, "How is she doing?"

I responded that she was doing great. I told her that her last day of preschool was the previous week and she had done great on her school performance. I also thanked her for all she had done thus far to allow me to witness that component in Paris' life.

The main topic I wanted to discuss was the 1 percent of chromosome that was present within her bone marrow. Dr. Kramer explained that there currently is and has been for the past few bone marrow samples an extra piece/copy of chromosome 1Q. Chromosomes are divided into either P's and Q's. The cells looked normal; however there was just that 1 percent of the chromosome 1Q present within the bone marrow sample. She stated that she had never seen that particular chromosome present before. She added that Paris could have been born with it; however that was unlikely, as it had not been present in the previous samples. She added that it was most likely a change as a result of chemotherapy. The percentages that they tend to be cautious of are 25 percent as a precursor to leukemia, and chromosomes commonly associated with leukemia are 5, 7, 8, and 11Q.

On June 13, I received a call from a friend of mine who is also a cancer mom. We had always texted back and forth to check on each other, as I commonly do with other cancer moms who are in other states doing treatments with their children. My phone rang, and I saw her name appear on the screen. I contemplated answering it, as I could predict what the phone call would be about. I let it ring four times knowing on the fifth ring it would go to my voicemail. I picked it up and immediately heard her screaming and crying. I immediately knew what had happened. She screamed, "Lauren, my baby girl is gone forever...forever Lauren." All I could do was listen to the chaos, and all I could say was, "I'm so sorry." Again it was another child that I had the pleasure of meeting, taken too soon and unfairly. I thought to myself, I could be the one making this phone call to someone, I'm not exempt.

On June 17 we went to the pediatrician to receive Paris' first set of the DtaP, HIB, IPV, and Prevnar vaccinations. I told Paris that we were at the doctor's office for a checkup and that she needed to get a little pinch in the arm to stay healthy. As soon as she saw the nurse enter with the tray of four needles she began to scream, "I'm scared! No mommy!" and began to thrash, twist, and turn to get away. I held her down forcing her to hold still, and the nurse poked her quickly giving her two of the shots in her left arm. We then switched to the right arm taking a little break. Her valiant attempt to fight to get away made her so sweaty. As the nurse approached her again she repeatedly cried, "I want my daddy." Again, holding her down, as she fought even harder than the first time since she knew what to expect, the nurse poked the remaining two shots in the right arm and we were done. The nurse left and all Paris kept saying was, "Mommy rock me, rock me. I'm so sad." I brought her favorite character bandages, which helped, and afterward I took her to the candy shop, where we splurged on whatever candy she wanted.

Chapter 34: Preparing for London

Ralph and Paris traveled to New York in July for the routine set of three-month scans. They would be gone only from July 25 to 28, God willing. It was supposed to be my turn to travel since I was off of work for the summer, but we had recently found out that I was pregnant, which greatly impacted my ability to go on the trips. The MIBG injection contains radioactive material, which is very dangerous for anyone who is pregnant. The hospital gave us a card that said, "The named child has had a procedure in nuclear medicine; measureable levels of radioactivity may be detected until 8/2/11." From the time of injection, which was July 26, until August 2, a total of eight days, she had the potential to give off radiation.

The less frequently you get scans, the harder it becomes because spending less time at the hospital helps your child resume a normal life for the most part. I think there was more pressure now because I potentially could get thrown back into the active lifestyle of treatment for someone who has cancer in a heartbeat, and I desperately wanted her to experience being a big sister and to enjoy that.

When Ralph and Paris were flying back, Ralph told Paris, "You did a great job in New York."

Paris looked at him and said, "Well, dad, I cried."

Ralph said, "It's okay that you cried. You still did a good job."

Paris added, "And remember, I did fight, too." Ralph simply laughed.

We discussed with the oncology team the possibility of us rotating scans between New York and our home hospital, as the travel back and forth every three months was getting to be quite costly. At times, the corporate flights did not travel at the same times as our scans.

Six months after her initial placement of growing rods, Paris underwent her second orthopedic surgery in September for Dr. Greyhack to adjust them. It was scheduled as an outpatient procedure, and as I understood it, Paris would be sedated and the surgery would be less invasive than the initial surgery. Paris went easily with the anesthesiologist, as he was a kid-friendly person. We thought that the procedure would last no more than a few hours; however they took her at 7:45 a.m. and didn't finish until noon. The orthopedic surgeon said he had to make the incision two-thirds or 8 inches larger than the initial cut to adjust the rods and make some minor adjustments to the hardware. That seemed pretty significant considering that Paris' spine was only 9 and a half inches in length.

After she awoke from the anesthesia, Paris ate light foods and looked at me and said, "Mommy, when the man with the little hat took me, he tried to put a mask on my face, and I covered my mouth like this," as she held her hands over her mouth to demonstrate. She proceeded by saying, "Mommy, I was so scared and I was calling for you, but you didn't come." I tried to explain that mommies were not allowed in the room and that this was just another time that she had to be brave in order to stay healthy.

After her recovery, Paris had to wear Pull Ups, which was a change from her character underwear. She was upset that she was back in the "squishy diapers," as she referred to them, but we explained that she had to wear them until her back healed again. She refused to take her pain medication. Even when we forced them, she threw them up, which made the situation even worse because then I really had to move her from her flat position. As she laid in her bed over those few days, she would call out that she had to go potty. We told her that for now she would have to go in her Pull Up since she was unable to sit upright. She squirmed and crossed her legs and stated, "Mommy, I have to go pee-pee. Please mommy, don't be mad, okay?"

These comments broke my heart, as I had to tell her that I wouldn't be upset and once her back healed she would be back on the potty. It was heartbreaking to watch and know that one day she was doing so well and the very next day she was in so much pain, a pain she didn't even expect to come, and was so confused as to why this happened.

September 10, 2011, marked the day that Paris had been stable for two years. We had been blessed during those two precious years, however, we never really forgot that in an instant we could be thrown right back into the cancer world. We never let this brief freedom take away the reality that childhood cancer is an epidemic, causing seven children to pass away every day.

Two days later, as I was giving Paris a bath, I noticed a pea-sized bump on the left side of her body, specifically located four fingers from her left nipple toward her armpit. As soon as I felt it, I feared the worst. I quickly finished the bath and called Ralph to feel it as well. At first he didn't feel anything and questioned if I had really felt anything or just thought I had felt something. I knew I did and found it quickly without trying to alarm Paris that I was frantically searching for this pea-sized bump. After I had located it, I showed Ralph specifically where it was, and he now had "that look" upon his face. He called my mom, and as he spoke to her, I quickly emailed Children's Memorial Hospital and Memorial Sloan-Kettering, hoping that Children's Memorial, our home hospital, could squeeze her in for an appointment.

After those emails, I began to feel sick, paranoid, and nauseous, and I began to panic. I walked up the first flight of stairs toward my bedroom and became consumed with the worst feeling of pain and dizziness as I approached the second flight. I'm not sure how exactly I made it to the bedroom doorway, but I remember grabbing ahold of it and feeling disorientated. I called for Ralph, as he was still downstairs. Then, unbeknownst to me, I fell face first onto the carpeted floor. Ralph heard the fall and ran upstairs, finding me face down and unresponsive. Mind you, I was pregnant. As he shook me awake, I didn't know where I was or how I had gotten there and then became engulfed with pain on the left side of my face, which was covered in a severe rug burn.

On September 13, 2011, I received a call from the team in Chicago saying there was an opening for a CT scan. Ralph, Paris, and I drove downtown, and the team assessed the bump. The team's impression was that Paris might possibly have a post-surgical lymph node rather than cancerous, however, based on her history, they needed to take precautionary measures to ensure it was not a relapse. The team ordered a CT scan for later in the afternoon, which unfortunately was canceled due to scheduling issues. It was rescheduled for Thursday, September 15, 2011. The next step was to further assess the results of the CT by ordering an MIBG scan for the following week.

The results indicated that the concerning bump was in fact just a reactive lymph node as a result of Paris being sick. All was well, and we were able to continue our three-month scan cycle in New York followed by three months of normalcy, in addition to preparing for Paris' new little sister, London.

I had many high-level/high-risk ultrasounds throughout the course of my pregnancy due to Paris' diagnosis. I had to go to the doctor many times, and often Paris would accompany me. I had to convince her that the appointments, which also required blood work, were not for her. As the doctor approached me, Paris began to scream "Don't hurt my mommy!" It was very admirable that she was trying to protect me from any type of perceived danger. Throughout all of my appointments I felt confident that London would be healthy. It was wonderful to see Paris so involved and so excited about becoming a big sister.

Ralph and I were very blessed to welcome another life into this world. When London was born on January 24, 2012, I constantly thought about how could I have one daughter who is perfectly healthy and another who is so sick? Paris is a wonderful big sister and instantaneously fell in love with London. It's a blessing to see them together. I have gotten a chance to see London through some of the milestones that I never got to experience with Paris, and in that respect I feel fortunate and like a first-time parent. At the same time, it's sometimes hard to watch London do some of the things that every child is supposed to do at a given milestone that I never got to experience with Paris. Watching her do it takes me right back to Paris' struggles.

Chapter 35: Feelings

Cancer affects the entire family. Siblings often take second place due to the ongoing attention that needs to be given to the child undergoing treatment. It is inevitable that the child who is diagnosed gets more attention than other siblings regardless of how fair you try to make it. Siblings are exposed to so much and go through so much as innocent bystanders. They have a great sense of compassion and character about them as they have been taught life lessons that some adults never learn.

Parents tend to feel robbed of things due to treatment. Overall the kids that have battled through it are okay with everything. It's the parents who seem to have trouble adjusting. Leftover scars, missing teeth, growth issues, hearing aids, thinning hair, cognitive issues, and physical disabilities will serve as a constant reminder to embrace every day, realizing that she or he is a survivor. As a parent, I hate what could occur from treatment, but it's the price Paris may pay to be a survivor.

My mom has pictures of me from Kiddieland, and when I took Paris, I saw the rides that I was once on. I put her in the same car that I sat in when I was younger, according to the photo. I was a bit nervous about putting her on the rides in fear that she would cry the whole time. As soon as we walked through the gate, her eyes lit up and she was glowing. She looked as if she didn't know what she wanted to ride first. I saw her light up, smiling from ear to ear and waving. Then I put her on the flying saucer and fighter jet rides that lifted up and down. She was in heaven. Her facial expression is permanently engraved in my head and on my heart. I have never seen her so happy from doing something. It makes me so happy that I was able to share that with her.

I felt guilty at times because I could not give Paris the things that I wanted to or control the situation. The path that we are on does not in any way, shape, or form match what I thought her life would be. I sometimes feel like I have failed her, even though I know that this situation is out of my control. Sometimes I feel victimized rather than in control.

It's a long, crazy, emotional, exhausting road that we always seem to battle. There are no easy answers. No disease affects these kids the same way. What works for one may not work for another. Treatment is always a gamble. Get second opinions. There are so many valuable doctors and treatment plans always on the horizon. Just remember not to question, look back on, or second guess your decisions once you make them. You do what's right at the time with the information that you have at that moment. Sometimes there's no time to think about it; you just have to do. You're in a whole new world now, and you will have to learn to adapt to it and learn to be part of it. Things will always get better with time.

A friend once posted, "You can't let the punches knock you down. You can be heartbroken but not defeated."

I BELIEVE POEM
I took a few excerpts from a poem entitled I believe that were memorable for me. The author is unknown.

> I Believe...
> That you should always leave loved ones with
> Loving words. It may be the last time you see them...
> I Believe...
> That you can keep going long after you think you can't.
> I Believe...
> That heroes are the people who do what has to be done when it
> Needs to be done, regardless of the consequences.
> I Believe...
> That maturity has more to do with what types of experiences
> You've had and what you've learned from them and less to do
> With how Many birthdays you've celebrated.

I Believe...
Two people can look at the exact same
Thing and see something totally different.
I Believe...
That your life can be changed in a matter of
Hours by people who don't even know you.
I Believe....
That even when you think you have no more to give,
When a friend cries out to you –
You will find the strength to help.
I Believe...
That credentials on the wall do not make you a decent human
Being.
I Believe...
That the people you care about most in life are taken from you
Too soon.
I Believe…
The happiest of people don't necessarily have the best of
Everything;
They just make the most of everything

Chapter 36: My Journey with Cancer

In May 2012, Ralph and Paris went to New York for an entire work-up, consisting of a brain/spine MRI, MIBG injection and scan, and bone marrow aspirations. Paris was now 5 years old, and this was the first time that they would be able to collect her urine sample without having to place a catheter while she was sedated. As Ralph and Paris were resting to prepare for the following day of scans, he heard her whispering in her bed. He asked her what she was doing.

She responded "praying to God."

Ralph asked her what she was asking him. She said that she asked him to "protect my IV and make it feel better."

Ralph asked her if she talks to God a lot, and she said, "All the time, and he answers me." Again her scans remained stable.

***

As I was getting Paris ready for bed on June 6, she started whining and requested to lay down with me in my bed. Ralph was downstairs watching the basketball game, so I let her snuggle with me. Unbeknownst to her, I had a doctor appointment the next day. As I told her good night, she stated completely unprompted, "Mommy you're going to go to heaven first because if I go you would miss me too much." She continued by saying, "The soldiers came to get me, but God made them bring me back," and didn't further explain with my prompting. She simply said, "I'm tired mom. Goodnight."

On June 7, 2012, I heard the words, "You have cancer," and they were specifically addressed to me. Automatically a million thoughts entered my head, but the most predominant thoughts focused around Paris and London. At first, I thought how does this happen? I'm supposed to remain healthy to take care of my child with cancer, but I now am part of the cancer world, fighting the battle that my daughter has been fighting for the past four years. My fear was if I would be blessed to live long enough to see my oldest daughter grow and beat cancer and would I survive long enough for my youngest daughter to even know who I was.

It began when I felt a lump in my right breast in 2002 and then again in 2008. Throughout that time I had it routinely checked, and the results had always come back benign as cysts. These small clusters of benign cysts would arise and disappear when I became stressed, around the time of my menstrual cycle, or when I was pregnant, but there was never a concern for malignancy.

After London was born, I noticed a change in the spot they had always been and decided to schedule an ultrasound appointment. That turned into a mammogram, followed by a needle biopsy. My mom, Paris, and London went with me to the appointment at Northwestern Memorial Hospital. As I waited with the hospital gown on, Paris asked, "Mommy, are you ok?"

I said, "Yes. I just needed to do some scans like you."

She said, "Well, it looks like you're having another baby," which made me chuckle.

As the mammogram imagining was being conducted, I immediately saw the white clusters appear on the screen and listened as the tech said, "I'll be right back." All of us cancer moms have been well educated on what happens next. I knew undoubtedly what the next words were going to be. I sat and prepared myself for the doctor to return to deliver me the news, and I just prayed that the cancer would not be life threatening.

Instantaneously, I was reliving the event from November 29, 2007, except this time I was the patient awaiting the news and was no longer naive or unfamiliar as I once was. The events in my past had "fortunately" hardened me to almost not be as emotional and disconnected to the new diagnosis, as I had adopted the motto, "Just do rather than just feel."

The doctor entered the room and said, "After reviewing the image, the area looks concerning. Therefore, I'd like to do a needle biopsy."
As the doctor conducted the needle biopsy, I directly asked, "So when the samples come back positive, what will the plan be?"

She said, "Let's not jump to conclusions," however; I already knew I had cancer cells within my body. I asked again.

Her response was, "It looks concerning, which is why we are doing the biopsy."

I then inquired persistently. "I just need to know the options."

She then began to explain that the area where the lump was located – the inner quadrant is an atypical area for breast cancer. Assuming it came back positive; the doctor said that I could either have a lumpectomy, which would remove the designated area, followed by radiation treatment. However, a buildup of scar tissue from radiation could hide potential unforeseen spots in the future, not to mention that radiation has a risk of secondary cancers. Alternatively, I could opt to have a mastectomy, which would remove the entire breast, eliminating radiation, and would significantly decrease my chances of recurrence and increase survival rates.

There were many factors to consider, however my first priority was Paris and my second was London, so whatever measure needed to be taken for them was what I was planning to have done. Paris' situation had prepared me quite well to ask the necessary questions and understand the process, so I was not feeling new to the cancer world again. That gave me a sense of comfort, and I was able to proceed with the right frame of mind.

I contacted Ralph, and his reaction was truly emotional. He was now faced with the reality of having two people that he loves – his daughter and his wife – deal with cancer. Ralph's initial reaction was the feeling of unfairness, questioning this as a punishment for something. After the initial shock, his reaction regarding options turned stronger, and he stated, "We are going to do whatever is necessary for you to see Paris and London grow up, and that's exactly the plan."

My oncologist team diagnosed me with ductal carcinoma, which is 2.4 centimeter, stage 2A grade 3 with invasive and noninvasive components. The results of the BRCA genetic component indicated that I do not have the BRCA 1 or 2 gene. They suggested a chemotherapy regiment, which I started on June 19, 2012. The treatment began with Adriamycin or Doxorubicin, nicknamed the red devil, which is commonly associated with heart damage, so I had to undergo echocardiograms that use sound waves to check how well my heart was functioning and pumping, just as Paris did throughout her journey. It also included cyclophosphamide, or Cytoxan, and Taxol once a week, every other week over a four-month span, followed by either a lumpectomy or mastectomy.

I went into the first appointment thinking, "I fight today so tomorrow I can survive." The most emotional part, as I had been told by many who have encountered this journey before, would be losing my hair 14 days after beginning chemotherapy. However, I have a 5 year old who has lost her hair four times during her short little lifetime and showed no complaint. I had to decide to accept this challenge and become mentally strong for what awaited me. I could and would embrace this journey and adopt the grace and strength shown by my daughter along with the countless children who face cancer on a daily basis.

Since I tested positive for HER 2, which indicates my cancer as an aggressive form, I would then be given Herceptin, an antibody treatment given once a month as outpatient for a year and then tamoxifen as a daily estrogen suppressant pill for 10 years since the tumor markers tested positive for being estrogen sensitive. I was faced with doing some of the exact chemotherapy drugs that Paris took from 9 days old to 2 years old.

Randomly one day, Paris said, "I hope I never get boobs." I was caught off guard and asked her why. Her reply was, "Well, mom, you know I already had cancer, and if I get boobs I don't need to get cancer again." I had to explain to her that her cancer was different than mine and that at this time she didn't have any bad cells in her body. Then I think, what a connection she made. What child thinks like that? What child should have to think like that?

I believe that anyone can do the unimaginable when faced with it. Anyone can do the impossible; you never know how strong you are until you're forced to be. People find their balance, and automatically instincts just kick in. Overall, I needed to remain positive and confident solely for Paris' sake. I needed to remember that this journey was only temporary. I needed to embrace the challenges that arose, knowing that there would be times that would be extremely difficult, both emotionally and physically, for me to face.

Every three months Paris underwent scans, and at any given time she was at risk for relapse or treatment-induced secondary cancers. It was my duty as her mother to show her that I could be brave, have strength, and overcome any situation that may seem destructive. I needed to show her that losing hair is simply that. That it doesn't define who you are as a person. That without hair is still beauty despite looks, stares, or comments. Confidence lies from within. Even when you look your best, there will always be someone who says you don't. I wanted to instill that Paris needs to be full of confidence and not let the unknown of others affect her. Although not the bonding experience I wanted to share with my daughter, I was accepting this challenge as a surreal experience that I would be able to feel exactly what she was unable to verbally express.

In the first few days after my diagnosis, I received an influx of "I'm sorry, I can't believe this is happening to you of all people," comments from my "normal" group of friends. I also received the "I'm gonna save the cliché shit, you know the drill, fight like hell, and kick cancer's ass" comments from my friends who have or who are dealing with cancer on a regular basis. It was interesting to hear two very different sets of motivational comments. I also kept hearing that God wouldn't give me more that I could handle. Even though I believed this, I wished that he wouldn't trust me so much.

The comment that took me most by surprise was when I was asked if I would feel like "less of a woman" by having the three main components representative of being a women being taken: my hair, breasts, and ability to reproduce. Even though those factors are sad and hard to adjust to, I was surprised that my response was quite simple: "I'm not defined by what I have or don't have. I'm defined by what I am blessed with and by how much I would sacrifice for my daughters and family."

I was embraced with heartfelt comments. A good friend told me, "Your strength is boundless, and you will get through this despite some days being harder than others. But Paris showed how much a child can endure, and now it's your turn to show her where she got her courage." Another good friend gave this perspective: why not me? God may be asking me to examine all of the reasons he had chosen me to endure this battle. I have a loving, strong, and supportive husband. I have already fought this battle with my daughter, who has shown thousands what bravery is. I have an incredible family and a network of friends that love and support me. Overall, until I am told that my options were slim or limited and we were faced with death as the only option, there were options. Some were better than others, but in the midst of things, I began to prioritize the importance of things. You're here to live until the day you die. Like I've said in the past, along Paris' treatment plan and journey since birth, as long as it's not Paris that has to endure the pain and suffering, I'll take the brunt of whatever comes my way in a heartbeat. During this journey, I would have to focus on the things that I could control and make the best out of the things that I couldn't.

Two months later, on August 22, Paris and Ralph left for New York for her three-month scan checkup, which consisted of brain and spine MRIs, MIBG injection and scan, and bone marrow aspirations. Since I got pregnant and was now newly diagnosed with breast cancer, Ralph had taken on the primary responsibility of accompanying her. He always did a phenomenal job. The results of these images indicated that Paris had been blessed with another three months of being stable.

***

On August 21, 2013, Dr. Kramer sent an e-mail to state that she was happy to report that Paris' scans look great and wanted me to consider a new possibility rather than continue to scan every three months. She said the team discussed Paris during their team meeting and felt that since she is this far out from her diagnosis, she only needs long-term follow-up care. This means no more scans/testing for neuroblastoma. She recommended that Paris be evaluated regularly for long-term effects from her treatment but was hopeful that neuroblastoma is not something to ever deal with again. My response was hesitant, as we had been scanning in New York every three months for the past four years. I was thinking that we would gradually move scans to every six months in either New York or Chicago now that Paris had proven she was able to complete all scans without the use of anesthesia. My main concern was a secondary cancer. I was very excited that the team felt hopeful and confident about Paris' health, but at the same time I felt conflicted at having reached this point.

Paris began her kindergarten experience on August 22, 2013. Part of me secretly didn't think I would see her reach this point, so to be able to experience it despite what she has endured was remarkable. Even though it had been an amazing experience thus far, it was also a realization of some challenges that await Paris. She was beginning to realize her limitations as she compared herself to her friends within the normal kindergarten setting. For her picture day, Paris wanted to wear "dress-up party shoes" to match her dress instead of her gym shoes with braces. She complained and said that she looked beautiful until people saw her feet. She said "these brace shoes don't even match!" She wanted to wear fancy shoes like her friends. She said, "I can't wait until I don't have to wear my braces anymore so I can wear sandals and pretty shoes." She also noticed that she doesn't move as fast as her peers in gym or at recess and that she had difficulty with her balance. She wanted to join gymnastics like her friends. She would become sad that she couldn't make large splashes during swim class. She was so sensitive she had started to cry about being "different" when she would tell me about her day. We would often have to point out and recognize her special talents and instill that it was okay to be different.

I would tell her, "When you get older, you are going to find that one special talent, that gift that God gave to only you." She was still noticeably frustrated at times but accepted her fate and carried on the best she can.

September 10, 2013, marked four years of Paris being stable.

Chapter 37: Appreciate

For cancer parents, the daily trials and tribulations that people face seem trivial to us as we are constantly battling for our children to get healthy, to simply see a smile on their face as they endure so much pain and wait for a cure to be found. Everyday life seems very trivial to us and is truly put into perspective when we think of the families that we have become close with who no longer have their children to hold and watch grow because they were so viciously taken from them. It makes you re-evaluate the things that frustrate and upset you. But again, this way of thinking is the normal for us. To others who have not been exposed to the everyday battle and suffering that we see on a regular basis, the so-called trivial things are very important because they have nothing to compare them to. If everyone for just one day actually got to witness a child in so much pain and in the hospital battling cancer, would the image be embedded so much in their mind that it would force them to change their way of thinking, their way of handling things, or would they be affected for the moment and then carry out their routine, walking away saying, "I'm so glad that's not me?" The bottom line is that people are affected when they are living it and breathing it every day. Other than that, people are just naturally consumed by their everyday problems and situations, which are seen as difficult for them.

Everyone before diagnosis had their problems that they thought were big. I would worry about money. Now in comparison, I would much rather deal with the problem of being broke compared to seeing your child sick. When bigger things come along, it makes you re-evaluate how you saw things before even though you thought those initial things were too big to handle in the first place. "You just don't know until you experience it." Everyone has significant events in their lives that shape who they are. I learn from this disease every day, and it truly forces me to value every minute, because we really are all in the position that we may not know what tomorrow may bring.

When in a normal situation, I believe that people really do take things for granted without even realizing it. Sure, you may say that you care about this and that, but there are few people that really take the time to make a difference in what they believe is important. If you're living in a perfect world, it is understandable that the everyday struggles of others may go unnoticed. If you're not living it, you may think about it, but it doesn't directly impact or affect you. You may make a comment or think about it for a minute, but then just naturally you go about your everyday personal struggles and everyday life. I understand because I did it. I saw the commercials for St. Jude and thought, "That is horrible," or "That's sad," but never in a million years did I think that would be my life. No one does. The opinion typically doesn't change until it happens to you, which forces you to begin to see things differently.

I hear about all the parents who need a break and time to themselves. It seems so frustrating to hear those things after you have dealt with a child who has a serious illness. You never want any time by yourself because you are so fearful that you won't get those moments back. I hear people say things negatively about their children or complain about something that they did or speak of needing a break from their child. I don't know, I guess everyone needs a break and time to themselves in the normal world. I probably would, too, if I wasn't in this situation, but you really begin to think about things differently when you have that normalcy taken away from you. You start to think you would never say something like that because every moment is treasured because it can so easily be taken away. You begin to want to scream at people and have them see things from your perspective, but that's difficult because everyone's belief, unless it happens to them, is, "that happens to other people, not me." Just imagine for a second not having your child with you permanently. Would you have looked back upon the times you needed time alone and regret it? Would you reflect on the comments you made toward your child, your frustration toward them for just being kids? Really appreciate moments spent with your children.

Open your eyes to truly appreciate life, because it can be taken from you in an instant. Being thankful, grateful, and appreciative of the little things that often go unnoticed seems to be a common theme for me. People get wrapped up in their everyday lives and miss the opportunity to really value the important things in life. Please take a minute out of your day and really be grateful for the life that you have, which ultimately revolves around health. Try to pinpoint the positive aspects and let them be stronger than the downfalls.

Sometimes I wonder when I will wake up from this nightmare. Then I look long and hard in the mirror, and I realize that this nightmare will continue even when I am wide awake.

I was at a restaurant in New York, and we were seated in the back area where it was not crowded, except for one older gentleman and his mother and another group of women. I began to hear the man make very loud noises and quickly noticed that he had Tourette's syndrome. He began to hit and scream, and it was obvious that people became uncomfortable. As people noticed this when the waiter tried to seat them, they quickly asked to be moved to another section. I paid attention to how people reacted and how his mother reacted. His mother never said anything to the reactions of others. She must have gotten used to it over the years. It made me reflect on how people may do things indirectly or directly and how it affects others. I thought to myself, if my life was just normal and Paris wasn't diagnosed with cancer, would I have reacted the same way as others? Having Paris diagnosed with cancer and being on the other side of the fence, I have been exposed to the stares of others; the random inappropriate comments regarding her use of the binky, her tantrums, her weight, her imperfect walking, which have made me feel like an outsider. I have learned to keep my opinions of others in place to help me stay grounded. I found at times that it's hard to feel good. As a parent with a child who has neuroblastoma, you need to remember that your world has changed and that you're not always going to feel good in it. There may be times when you have some really bad days.

My mother has always been the type of person that would bend over backward for anyone. I didn't think that she could ever bend anymore, but she has always been there, over countless nights and days, doing anything that I ask. I've also become closer with my sister during this journey. She is one person that I can truly count on no matter what. My sister got a tattoo of an African symbol that represented strength and bravery, and as she showed it to me, she told me about how she chose it because of me. She said that she feels that I am the strongest and bravest person she knows.

I began to subconsciously anticipate the special days as being the last days because you never know when cancer will decide to take over, fully taking away your future holidays. Therefore, you try to make everything perfect. Spending a lot of time worrying if this event is perfect causes a lot of arguments and stress, instead of just enjoying the moment and letting things happen. It gets difficult because you wonder if you will get the opportunity to have this moment again.

Once we were out of that cancer element, I would reflect on pictures in which, at the time, I thought that Paris looked good. Compared to our break and decent health, those pictures make her look very sick. When I look back on the pictures that captured her in active treatment, she looks devastating. When I'm not in the situation and am able to compare her appearance, it looks worse than what I actually thought at the time.

When I watch Paris and see her sing to songs, dance, read books, play with her toys, color, and watch TV, it just amazes me. She finds such joy in doing these things. She's happy and really does enjoy life. For Paris, the ouchies and pain are just a part of her life. She has been exposed to it since day 9, and she doesn't know any different. She doesn't know that there is a life without all of the complications and ouchies. When I watch her for those moments of just being a kid, I really absorb them. That is what she should be doing every day.

Every child is different and handles pain and treatment differently, but I have seen Paris go through the worst pain imaginable, chronic vomiting, rapid weight loss, lack of appetite, loss of hair, and overall a full body transformation from the child that I once knew at 9 days old into a child that you could never imagine, one with a physical appearance that you would never wish upon anyone. But through every obstacle, she continues to exhibit extreme strength, determination, and strong will. I often wonder how tall she would really be, how much she would weigh and what her hair would really look like if she didn't have to endure these challenges. Would she still be feisty, or would she be more timid and shy if she didn't have to always fight and be strong?

It's so difficult to process your child speaking in medical terms and repeating things that you never once thought they would be exposed to. Before each sedation, Paris has been conditioned to grab my face and say, "Mamma, no ouchie. Promise." What do I even say?

I agree, "Okay, no ouchie. Promise," knowing that she won't remember any of the scans afterward.

I feel like I'm always fighting time. Before bed, Paris asks me if she can do certain things the following day, and of course, whatever she asks, we do without hesitation or question because we realize how important time with our child is. But the thought does pass in my mind; please let her make it through the night so we can always fulfill her request for the morning. After our prayers I always tell her, as I tuck her in, how much I love her and that I'll see her when the sun comes up.

Her response is always, "Definitely."

I always remember that strength lies within and that life accompanied with every experience, whether good or bad, makes you stronger.

Chapter 38: Forever a Number

"Death leaves a heartache no one can heal. Love leaves a memory no one can steal."- Anonymous

I can't even write this section without tears building in my eyes because it's surreal and there is a possibility I can be on the other side of the coin at any given moment. I am not just writing about death in general. I'm writing about little children and families that I have grown close with over time. Ones that had the same cancer as Paris. We are not exempt from this.

When you enter this cancer world, you meet families either at the start of treatment, during relapse, during hospital stays, during treatment procedures, and during surgeries that unfortunately are on this journey with you. These people that you meet over time become your immediate family, even if the conversation is minimal. I always kept a record of whom I spoke with because I have always kept their child in my thoughts. Once you have a child with cancer, everyone you meet impacts you. The group of mothers and fathers that I began this journey with refer to each other as veterans. I also met some families through websites and have followed their stories. These people also become like an extended family because you genuinely care about their children as well.

In the network of families, as your family grows, you face the possibility that some children you encounter will pass, which becomes very difficult to process. There are so many great minds working together to find a cure for neuroblastoma. No parent should ever have to fathom the idea of death. I am saddened when I learn about how many children have to pass or be subject to potential treatments before a cure is found.

Sometimes I sit and think about all of the friends that we have met and grown to love. I think of the bond that we created, even if I had only met then a few times, due to the connection that we all share. I think of the friends who have lost a child.

I wrote a list of all of the friends that I have met, and then as I looked at the list again, I realized in just two short years, a great majority of the names on the list have passed away.

Some of our friends who have earned their wings are Eli, Anna, Ila, Reitza, Erin, Erik, Justin, Kylie, Ashlynn, Deyja, Gina, Anthony, Gabby, Tyler, Emmy, Mattie, Morgan, Liam, Ylaria, Jensen, Rowan, Sandra, Liam, Ryan, Aisy, Nick, Jake, Ester, Owen, Andrea, Coen, Onja, Jack, Pierce, Nathan, Talia...there unfortunately are just too many.

The book entitled *Swan in Heaven* says that people who are dying typically wait for their loved ones to be somewhere else before taking their last breath. They want to ensure that you are at peace before they pass. I believe souls have intentions. They have the obligation to teach and transform the habits, beliefs, and behaviors of others.

The first time I received the news that a child that we actually knew had passed, I thought to myself, I spoke to them, I hugged them, I knew them, they shared toys with Paris, I saw them laugh, and I saw them cry, and they all have the same disease. I experienced survivors guilt, realizing that my child who is still alive has had some of the very same treatments administered, knowing that the very same complications can arise. It's a very surreal moment because I came face to face with the realistic possibility that the same disease can take Paris in an instant, at any unexpected moment, without warning.

After a child's journey battling neuroblastoma ends, they are known to have earned their angel wings. I dread getting the messages through email entitled "another angel gets his/her wings." I noticed that parents indicated that their child has earned their wings by placing marks on the outside of their name – ^^*and inserting the child's name*^^.

When a child passes, you are faced with the reality of how permanent it is. Death is all around us, and life is full of bad things that could potentially happen. Every day should be considered a blessing. There are obstacles all around us and tragic things can occur at any given minute. When your child is no longer present with you in physical form, every little thing around you will trigger a memory of him or her. It doesn't ever really get easier. The typical person doesn't realize the impact losing a child has unless they have experienced it.

I once heard, "The journey with loss begins as the journey with cancer ends." You have daily distractions to keep your mind busy, but there is always an annual holiday, birthday, first day of school, or other event that triggers your memory along the way. Glances of items within the house, hearing something that someone says that's similar to a phrase your child commonly used, memories that filter your mind constantly, determining if you can find the strength to leave your house, glances of other children that may resemble him or her, receiving sympathy cards in the mail that trickle in afterwards, phone calls from nurse case managers to clarify information, calls from hospitals or collection agencies requesting payment, calls from pharmacies to refill prescriptions – all whom have not yet been informed of the passing – can bring instant feelings of despair. No matter how much time passes, it doesn't get easier, as memories are among us every day. The pain may lesson some days or may be masked by other daily life distractions, but it will never go away.

Hallmark introduced an ornament in 2010 as part of its collection entitled Always Remembered. It was the most beautiful representation of death to me. It was an oyster with a white pearl inside.

Everyone has the thought about their child being taken from them, and we all plead with God not to take them from us and to cure them, allowing them to outlive us. I can't even imagine losing a child. I can't personally speak of that. I just know that based on being so close to families who have lost a loved one that it is extremely difficult, and I hope that people eventually find peace over time. I found a poem entitled, "I Have a Place in Heaven" that for me gives a little comfort for the children that have been taken too early.

> Please don't sing a sad song for me, forget the grief and fear
> For I am in a perfect place, away from pain and tears.
> It's far away from hunger and hurt and want and pride
> I have a place in heaven with the Master by my side.
> My life on Earth was very good as Earthly life can go
> But paradise is so much more than anyone can know.

A friend of mine named Michelle lost her child and shared this with me: "The weight of grief is always the same, but if you carry it every day, it gets easier to lift." I have heard stories of people who have sought out medians, and I do believe in that. I think it is important to find answers to the unknown with a reputable source to ensure that your child is at peace.

The world decides when your suffering should end and when you should return back to the normal life. People will say, "Don't you feel enough time has passed?" or "It's time to go on with life." To respond to the factor of time, I came across a poem entitled, "The Path."

> This is my path. It was not a path of my choice, but a path that I must walk with intention. It is a journey through grief that takes time. Every cell in my body aches and longs to be with my beloved child.
>
> I may be impatient, distracted, frustrated and unfocused. I may get angry more easily, or I may seem hopeless. I will shed many many tears. I won't smile as often as my old self. Smiling hurts now. Most everything hurts some days, even breathing.
>
> But please just sit beside me. Say nothing. Do not offer me a cure, or a pill, or a word or a potion. Witness my suffering and don't turn away from me.

Please, self, be gentle with me too. I will not ever get over it so please do not urge me down that path. Even if it seems I am having a good day, maybe I am even able to smile for a moment; the pain is just beneath the surface of my skin.

Some days I feel paralyzed. My chest has a nearly constant sinking pain, and sometimes I feel as if I will explode from grief. This is affecting me as a woman, a mother, a human being. It affects every aspect of me; spiritually, physically, mentally, and emotionally. I barely recognize myself in the mirror anymore.

Remember that grief is as personal to each individual as a fingerprint. Don't tell me how I should or shouldn't be doing it or that I should or shouldn't feel better by now. Don't tell me what's wrong or right. I'm doing it my way, in my time. If I am to survive this, I must do what is best for me. Surviving this means seeing life's meaning change and evolve.

What I knew to be true or absolute or real or fair about the world has been challenged, so I'm finding my way, moment to moment in this new place. Things that once seemed important to me are barely thoughts any longer. I notice life's suffering more – hungry children, the homeless and the destitute, a mother's harsh voice toward her young child or that of an elderly person struggling with the door.

So many things I now struggle to understand. Don't tell me that God has a plan for me. This, my friend, is between me and my God. Those platitudes seem far too easy to slip from the mouths of those who tuck their own children into a safe warm bed at night. Can you begin to imagine your own child, flesh of your flesh, lying lifeless in a casket, when goodbye means you'll never see them on this Earth again? Grieving mothers and fathers and grandparents and siblings won't wake up one day with everything okay and life back to normal. I have a new normal now. Oh, perhaps as time passes, I will discover new meanings and new insights about what my child's death means to me. Perhaps, one day, when I am very, very old, I will say that time has truly helped to heal my broken heart. But always remember that not a second of any minute of any hour of any day passes when I am not aware of the presence of his absence, no matter how many years lurk over my shoulder. Love never dies.

There is another poem entitled, "Don't Tell Me."

Please don't tell me you know how I feel unless you have lost your child too.

Please don't tell me my broken heart will heal, because it's just not true.

Please don't tell me my child is in a better place, though it is true I want her here with me.

Don't tell me that one day I'll hear her voice, see her face, beyond today I cannot see.

Don't tell me it's time to move on, because I cannot.

Don't tell me it's time to face the fact that she is gone, because denial is something I can't stop.

Don't tell me to be thankful for the time that I had, because I wanted more.

Don't tell me when I am my old self you will be glad. I'll never be as I was before

What you can tell me is you will be here for me, that you will listen when I talk about my child.

You can share with me your precious memories, you can cry with me for a while.

And please do not hesitate to say her name, because it is something I long to hear everyday.

Friend please realize that I can never be the same.

A friend of mine posted, "Please don't judge me now or think that I am behaving strangely. Remember, I am grieving. I may be in shock, I may feel afraid, I may feel deep rage, I may feel guilty, but above all

I feel hurt. I'm experiencing pain unlike I've ever felt before. Don't worry if you think I'm getting better and then suddenly slip backward. Grief makes me behave this way at times. Please don't tell me you know how I feel or that it's time to get on with my life."

Always remember that while it may be a great day for you, it is a horrific day for others. At this moment, parents are making the most difficult decisions in the world, ones that are unimaginable, having thoughts that should never have to pass through the minds of parents – to stop treatment and let their child be at peace.

I have known families having to make the decision to end treatment, the decision to not be selfish, to allow their child not to suffer anymore and be free from this horrific disease. But then to lose the most important thing to them? This is not fair. No parent should ever have to make decisions about their child's life at such a young age. These are not the decisions that a parent should ever have to face or make for their children. It is extremely difficult to decide on the type of burial for your child. There is debate amongst traditional burial and cremation. A child's casket can range from 18 inches to 5 feet. There are funeral homes out there, such as Enea Family located in New York that adjust the price of children's caskets to a sliding scale or simply do not charge. Many families bury their child; however I often hear that it becomes difficult to visit the grave site on a regular basis as time passes, which causes feelings of guilt. Consider the fact of what if you should move out of your current state or location? You may be one that believes the soul travels with you, which may be comforting if time constraints limit physically going to a cemetery. Other individuals choose to cremate so that the remains can be present with the family at all times. It's a personal decision, and everyone has to do what is best for them.

Another close friend of ours passed away close to Halloween, and his mother asked how could she celebrate the holidays without him? Someone had suggested that for Halloween a white pumpkin be used in place of the traditional orange pumpkins in honor of that child.

Families often start foundations or nonprofit organizations after or during their children's journey and as part of the healing process, with the goal of helping others, both financially and emotionally, who are in similar situations.

What do you do when your child's friend passes away from neuroblastoma? The easy answer is that no parent should ever have to tell their child that their little friend has passed away, let alone from the same disease that their little bodies carry. It's an individual decision, and as parents you know your child the best and you reserve your own right to decide what information your child can emotionally handle. In my opinion, there are many factors to consider before sharing that type of information, such as the age of the child and timing regarding his or her own treatment, considering that he or she, too, has the same disease. Paris understands the concept of death, as we have explained when someone passes they become angels in heaven. I personally never tell Paris when one of our little friends pass. When she mentions a friend from New York, I always say I'm sure he or she is enjoying a very healthy life right now.

My mind was cluttered with thoughts as so many close friends earned their wings after battling neuroblastoma. How do you sit with your child on hospice knowing that she will pass? How do you make peace with that other than to know that your child will no longer suffer? How do you go on with life without part of you? After speaking with some people regarding the loss of their children, they stated that they found comfort in the thought that "the chains of cancer kept them here, and now they are free, now they are cancer free forever." Hearing them look at their children's passing from that perspective for just a moment, despite their hurt and personal pain, was amazing.

One of my friends posted this story on her website after her sons passing.

"The Brave Little Soul," written by John Alessi.

You don't understand how traumatic it is unless you are faced with losing your child. I know people who have lost a child in utero or upon birth, and for those families, I feel sad. In any instance it's horrible to lose a child. I feel like it's even harder to lose a child once you have gotten to know their personality, and then you're faced with the possibility of losing your child after getting to know them. It is very difficult because you have formed a bond with them. I have created a relationship with my daughter, and the thought of losing that bond is very heartbreaking.

A friend once said, as she reflected on the recent passing of her son, "Every day without you is a day closer to holding you."

I have wondered what it would be like to lose a child since many other parents who battle neuroblastoma have lost their little ones along the way. I began to think how do they handle watching other children play, celebrating holidays and Mother's Day, responding to questions like, "Do you have children?" or "How do you go about your life when your child has been taken away from you?" I wonder how could I ever fathom or deal with a situation like this, and the first thought that comes to mind is, "Wait, I never thought I could handle dealing with a child who was diagnosed with cancer." It's when you're not faced with situations that you can't bear to think of how you would ever deal with them, but when you're faced with them, you seem somehow to manage even though it is extremely painful. It's never out of your mind, and you think about it every day, but you manage and you force yourself to continue on – eventually.

I came across a poem written by an unknown author:

> I thought of you and closed my eyes and prayed to God today,
> I asked "What makes a Mother?" and I know I heard him say:
>
> "A Mother has a baby, this we know is true." But, God, can
> you be a Mother when your baby's not with you?"

"Yes, you can" he replied with confidence in his voice. I have given many women babies, when they leave – it is not their choice.

Some I send for a lifetime and others for a day. And some I send to feel your womb, but there's no need to stay.

I just don't understand this God, I want my baby here!

He took a breath and cleared his throat and then I saw a tear. I wish I could show you what your child is doing today. If you could see your child smile with other children and say:

"We go to Earth to learn our lessons of love and life and fear, My Mommy loved me so much I got to come straight here. I feel so lucky to have a Mom who had so much love for me, I learned my lessons very quickly and my Mommy set me free."

"I miss my Mommy oh so much, but I visit her each day. When she goes to sleep, on her pillow is where I lay. I stroke her hair and kiss her cheek and whispers in her ear, Mommy, don't be sad, I'm your baby and I am here."

So you see, my dear sweet one, your child is okay. Your baby is here in my home and this is where she'll stay. She'll wait for you with me until your own lessons are through. And on the day you come, she'll be at the gates for you.

So now you see what makes a Mother, It's the feeling in your heart.
It's the love you had so much of right from the very start.

Though some on Earth may not realize until their time is done, remember all the love you have and know that you are A Very Special Mom.

I have known families who have been victims of medical identity theft, a scam on cancer patients. Predators will take the child's identity by gaining access to his or her social security numbers documented on medical records or other medical forms. Families who have had children that have passed have had complications filing their taxes and claiming their ill or deceased child as a dependent. People target the obituaries, target social media or hackers break into computer systems where social security numbers are kept. These children are victims of so many other unfortunate circumstances that identity theft should be the last thing they have to worry about.

In addition to losing a child to cancer, I have had a handful of cancer moms that I have personally known throughout this journey choose to end their own lives after the passing of their child. The pain of not having their child in the physical world becomes too unbearable, and without their child, life becomes pointless despite the fact that there may be other children involved. They cannot move on. I cannot judge anyone for their choices. I have not been in the position to feel that type of pain.

I have also known some cancer moms who have gone through severe post-traumatic stress syndrome and unimaginable mental breakdowns compiled with many of life's additional obstacles, and to them, at the moment, the challenges seem to never end, to the point where they see absolutely no light at the end of the tunnel. To the point where they put their own children, ones that have been battling cancer, ones that they so desperately have tried every remedy to save, in harm's way to abruptly end the battle with cancer and all the factors that accompany it, including their own life. I have not fallen victim to mental health issues, however I do know it's a serious disease that needs to be carefully monitored by women who are undergoing the role of a cancer parent. The consequences of mental health disorders not being carefully monitored has been known to have horrendous consequences to innocent victims.

Appendix 1: Medications

I wanted to create a list of the commonly used medications Paris had to take throughout her treatment plan.

Enfamil Enfalyte, natural light cherry flavor: Oral electrolyte solution that replaces the fluids and electrolytes commonly lost after diarrhea or vomiting

Ondansetron (Zofran): 2.5 mls every 8 hours to control nausea and vomiting

Ranitidine HCI Syrup: 0.46 ml every 4 hours to control nausea and vomiting

Dexamethasone (Decadron), oral solution

HydrOXYzine HCI (Vistaril) syrup: 3mg every 4 hours to control nausea, vomiting, hives and itching, usually after 3F8 or 8H9

Tylenol: Every 4 hours to prevent or control fever

Neomycin Sulfate

Lactulose Solution: 1 teaspoon needed for constipation

Liothyronine Sodium Tablets: 1 tablet given once daily

Sennoside A and B: 2 ml at bedtime

Docusate Sodium: 2ml by mouth daily

OxyCODONE HCI: Maximum dose 4.2ml every 4 hours for pain

HYDROmorphone HCI: Maximum dose 2.4ml per 24 hours for pain after IV3F8

Accutane (isotretinoin), an acne medicine developed in the 1980s, has been a treatment option for children with neuroblastoma. Also known as 13 cis retinoic acid, the drug is a very high dose vitamin A supplement. In a phase 3 trial, Accutane has been shown to prevent some children from relapsing. It is said to increase survival by 5 to 10 percent. Our trial through Sloan-Kettering planned for five cycles of Temodar and then Accutane, as the treatment plan usually consists of six months in between Temodar or up to 2 years post-chemo.

Some parents will pinch or cut the end of the gel capsule pill with tweezers or surgical scissors while wearing surgical gloves and use new pliers, cleaned thoroughly each time, to squeeze the yellow liquid onto a spoonful of fatty foods such as whipped cream, chocolate syrup, chocolate pudding, peanut butter, cheese grits, ice cream, or yogurt or into a yogurt drink, or they will wrap the entire pill into a gummy fruit roll up. You want to be careful that you do not tamper with foods that they favor so you don't risk them becoming resistant to them.

Children respond to Accutane differently. Some parents call it one of the most difficult treatments to endure. Side effects include dry, peeling, or chapped skin, mood swings, and/or uncontrollable tantrums. Parents have said that reevaluating the recommended dose tends to help with the behavior.

Many people have debated the use of Accutane. The FDA pulled it from the U.S. market in 2009 due to potentially dangerous side effects, including inflammatory bowel disease (IBD). Ralph and I made the difficult decision not to participate in the Accutane part of treatment after Paris completed 210 days of Temodar.

Catecholamines are substances within the body that derive from the amino acid tyrosine and act as hormones. The term represents the hormones that are commonly released: dopamine, spinephrine, and norepinephrine. Neuroblastoma tumors can cause increased levels of catecholamines to be secreted. This can cause the heart rate to increase, blood pressure to rise, and breathing to quicken as a response to stress, certain drugs, or food. The Vanillylmandelic acid (VMA) levels and Homovanillic acid (HVA) are measured during a urine collection test to determine the amounts of urinary catecholamines within the body. Certain foods increase urinary catecholamines such as coffee, tea, bananas, chocolate, most citrus fruits, pineapples, orange juice, tomatoes, plums, eggplant, avocado, kiwi, yogurt, licorice, walnuts, tea, and natural vanilla/vanilla-containing products. The following drugs can also increase catecholamine measurements: over-the-counter cold medicines that contain acetaminophen, such as Tylenol, levodopa, lithium, aminophylline, chloral hydrate, clonidine, disulfiram, erythromycin, insulin, methenamine, methyldopa, quinidine, reserpine, guaifenesin, and tetracyclines. It is recommended that these items be avoided several days (24 to 48 hours) prior to the tests.

Appendix 2: Resources

I spent countless hours researching information regarding neuroblastoma on the internet. It became my new obsession. I found myself becoming involved with organizations and fundraising efforts and networking with other parents who were also battling the disease. Due to Paris' extreme young age at the time the disease presented itself, I found that people would contact me as they stumbled upon Paris' website asking me questions or advice. I became friends with parents who were very involved. I became a member of online support groups. I almost felt like I became an expert in the field and had become someone else's angel at their time of need.

I believe in the cause and the fight for hope, and I figured that I would dedicate myself to any aspect surrounding neuroblastoma that needed my help. Many families, who have had children with neuroblastoma or other types of chronic illnesses, have started nonprofit organizations using a 501(c)3 account. In the event that their child passes, they may take what was donated and turn it into a funding source to aide other families who are currently facing hardships due to the cost of treatment.

Organizations

The Band of Parents is a nonprofit organization formed in 2007 by a group of parents who have or have had children diagnosed with neuroblastoma that have banded together to aide research in attempts to find a cure. It's difficult to provide research for children with neuroblastoma simply because of the limited number who are diagnosed each year, therefore funding for a cure is limited. The Band of Parents donates 100 percent of donations received to the team at Memorial Sloan-Kettering for innovative research. Humanized 3F8 is the first drug to be fully funded by the Band of Parents. Band of Parents and the neuroblastoma list serve have been very resourceful tools for me. I am privileged to be part of them. They are places

where questions can be answered and concerns, fears, and expressions of gratitude and happiness can be expressed or where you can just vent when the day seems extremely hard for both you and your child. Not everyone has access to these resources nor do they know about them, which is why I felt obligated to write this book so others may have the same outlet that I was given during the very difficult times of this journey.
www.bandofparents.org

The National Cancer Institute provides resources to individuals facing cancer. www.cancer.gov

The American Cancer Society provides resources to individuals facing cancer. www.cancer.org

The American Brain Tumor Association provides resources to individuals facing cancer.
www.abta.org

The National Children's Cancer Society (NCCS) mission is to improve the quality of life of children with cancer and serve as a financial, emotional and educational resource to families.
www.thenccs.org

Arms Wide Open for Childhood Cancer Foundation was started by Dena, our friend who we met in New York, after her son Billy was diagnosed with neuroblastoma. The nonprofit organization's primary focus is to raise funds for current treatment and alternative therapies. Dena has written a book entitled *No Retreat No Surrender* as a means of support for parents.
www.awoccf.org

The Children's Neuroblastoma Cancer Foundation (CNCF), hosted by Pat Tullungen, is committed to finding a cure for neuroblastoma. Our dear friend Kenna is vice president of this organization, which provides families with a wealth of information and resources.

www.cncfhope.org or www.cncf-childcancer.org

The Candlelighters Childhood Cancer Foundation is a nonprofit charitable organization dedicated to childhood cancer and supports the needs of families facing childhood cancer. The belief is that "kids can't fight cancer alone."
www.acco.org

Bear Necessities, currently Bear Hugs, established by Kathleen Casey in honor of her son Barrett "Bear," who passed away from neuroblastoma, provides small miracles for children under the age of 2, up to $500. This national 501(c)3 organization allowed Paris to celebrate her second birthday, since we were unable to celebrate her first due to treatment. Can you imagine being a first-time mother and missing your daughter's first birthday because you are in the hospital fighting for her life? Every mother wants to plan an extravagant birthday party for their child, but a medical emergency takes priority and can shatter the dreams of watching your child blow out her birthday candles for the first time. I promised myself the next time she felt healthy, we would celebrate in an extreme fashion, and Bear Hugs and Nelli Rose helped accomplish that dream.
www.bearnecessities.org

All Kids Health Care Insurance is a governed program that provides health care to children of Illinois.
www.allkids.com

The Illinois the Division of Specialized Care for Children of DuPage (DSCC) is through the University of Illinois at Chicago. This agency helps children who have special health care needs and provides care coordination. The agency found Paris' condition eligible and therefore provided her with diagnostic testing and assistance finding medical care. It works in collaboration with All Kids Insurance of Illinois, assists families with finding resources, works in collaboration in developing a plan for the future and maintains communication between doctors, specialists, and schools.

www.uic.edu/hsc/dscc

Kids V Cancer, founded in 2009 and created in honor of Jacob, promotes pediatric cancer research by identifying structural impediments at key junctures in the research process – new drugs, tissue donation, and access to funding – and developing strategies to use them.
www.kidsvcancer.org

Travel Assistance

Corporate Angel Network is a nonprofit corporation that flies patients to recognized treatment centers if there are empty seats available on either commercial airlines or corporate jets. I personally worked with many representatives from this organization. This charity works with families to coordinate travel plans.
1-866-328-1313.
info@corporateangelnetwork.org
www.corpangelnetwork.org

Miracle Flights for Kids in Nevada offers free commercial flights to the patient and charges $50.00 for one accompanying parent round trip to wherever the patient needs to go for treatment.
1-702-261-0494
www.miracleflights.org

Midwest Express Miracle Miles is based out of Wisconsin and offers one free flight to patients and then discounted flights afterwards.
1-414-570-3644

Angel Flight, a nonprofit operating out of Oklahoma, consists of pilots that dedicate their time to transport families with medical needs at no cost.
1-918-749-8992
www.angelflight.com

Air Charity Network is a nonprofit organization consisting of pilots that volunteer their time to transport patients to and from medical facilities at no cost.
www.aircharitynetwork.org

Air Star is an Arizona-based company that provides medical flights to patients on a discounted basis.
www.airstararizona.com

Children's Flight of Hope is a North Carolina–based organization that provides private medical air transportation to and from medical facilities throughout the Eastern United States at no cost.
www.childrensflightofhope.org

FOOTPRINTS in the Sky is a nonprofit organization based out of Denver that provides flights to patients throughout the United States to medical facilities at no cost.
1-303-799-0461
www.footprintsflights.org

Mercy Medical Air Lift is a charitable medical transportation system that is available for patients located in Virginia Beach.
1-800-296-1217
www.mercymedical.org

Sky Hope is located in Georgetown, Texas, and uses business aviation for small and large scale emergencies
1-561-714-30-70
www.sky-hope.org

National Patient Travel Center is a hotline available 24/7 that provides information about all forms of charitable long distance medical transportation.
1-800-296-1217
www.patienttravel.org

Life Line Pilots is a nonprofit organization that provides medical transportation on a small (4 to 6 person) private aircraft at no cost.
1-309-697-6865
www.lifelinepilots.org

Operation Lift Off is a nonprofit organization based out of St. Louis that provides air transportation for patients to specialized care or treatment centers. It also provides "special trips" for children with a life-threatening or serious illness or "group trips" for teenagers who are facing the same type of cancer or illness.
www.operationliftoff.org

Angel Bus provides long-distance ground bus transportation to patients at no cost.
1-757-333-0084
www.angel-bus.org

Housing Assistance

Ronald McDonald House Charities provides housing for families whose children are being treated in hospitals in every state. An act as simple as pulling off and saving the pop tops found on any aluminum cans can help raise money for the Ronald McDonald house, which houses children and families undergoing medical treatment. Approximately 4,175 pop tops equal $1.75. It is important to remember Margaret Mead's quote, "Never doubt that a small group of thoughtful committed citizens can change the world. Indeed it is the only thing that ever has."
www.rmhc.com

Wish Fulfillment Organizations
Make-A-Wish is the most well-known organization to fulfill a wish for a child having any chronic life-threatening illness. It grants wishes to patients between the ages of 2 and a half and 18 years old. I never thought that I would be receiving a Make-A-Wish packet in the mail

addressed to my daughter. I opened the envelope and thought to myself, "I'm not reading this solely for information. I'm reading this, and it is actually directed specifically to me." It was purely my lack of awareness, but I was always under the impression that the Make-A-Wish Foundation granted wishes to children who were near the point of passing, providing them with their last wish, something very special to them. However this is not the case. Children are able to obtain their wish before or during treatment or after remission.
www.wish.org

Children's Wish Foundation International
www.childrenswish.org

Cancer Kiss My Cooley (CKMC)
www.cancerkissmycooley.org

Dream Factory
www.dreamfactoryinc.org

Give Kids the World
www.gktw.org

Memories of Love
www.memoriesoflove.org

Western Wishes Foundation
www.westernwishes.org

Benefit4kids Outdoor Wish
21660 23 Mile Road
Macomb, MI 48044
www.B4K.org

Financial Assistance Organizations

As of April 2012, Social Security Disability, under the Compassion Allowances Initiative, announced 52 newly covered conditions, now including childhood neuroblastoma. With the newly added neurological disorders, cancers and rare diseases, the Compassion Allowance program fast-tracks disability decisions to be made within days rather than months or years. Contacting the social worker at the specific treatment facility can be a valuable resource toward obtaining financial assistance.
www.socialsecurity.gov/compassionateallowances

Miracles from Mia, a nonprofit organization, was developed by Georgianna Clements after the passing of her daughter Mia, who was diagnosed with Multi-Dysplastic Kidney Disease (MDK). The mission of her organization is to provide families of chronically ill children who reside in Illinois with financial and emotional support.
www.miraclesfrommia.org

Pennies for Penny provides financial assistance in various forms to families with a child battling neuroblastoma.
www.pennies4penny.org

Just In Time-Neuroblastoma Foundation, Inc., provides financial assistance to families located in Colorado.
www.justintimenbf.org

Sports for Kids is an organization designed to assist physically and/or emotionally challenged children through sports-related fundraisers. The proceeds raised are used to assist families with financial expenses for medical equipment.
www.sportsforkids.org

Local branches of the American Red Cross provide families with help paying electric and heating bills.

Life Beyond Cancer is an organization that was formed with a mission of helping cancer patients with bills and expenses such as rent, mortgage, food, car payments, car insurance and utility bills. www.lifebeyondcancer.org

Give Forward is a website that enables people to solicit financial help for medical expenses. www.giveforward.com

Go Fund Me helps families raise money for medical expenses. www.gofundme.com

Lifting Spirits Resources

Imerman Angels founded by Jonny Imerman, a cancer survivor himself, is an organization that provides families the opportunity to be paired with survivors of similar cancers. The main purpose is to share stories, words of encouragement, and hope. www.immermanangels.org

Alex's Lemonade Stand Foundation's motto is, "When life gives you lemons, make lemonade." It was founded by Alexandra "Alex," who was diagnosed with cancer and decided to raise money to find a cure. In one day, she raised $2,000. Her memory continues through lemonade stands all over the United States. The organization has been featured in *People Magazine,* which exposed people to the reality of childhood cancer. www.alexslemonade.org

Catie Hoch Foundation of Clifton Park, New York, was founded in memory of Catie and is dedicated to assisting families with the financial burden that accompanies children with neuroblastoma. www.catiehochfoundation.org

The late Anna O'Connor founder of Anna's Hope is a 501(c)3 charitable foundation dedicated to raising awareness and money for research into the cure for neuroblastoma.
www.annabanana.org

Cookies for Cancer was established and founded by Gretchen, who is a personal friend of ours. She was inspired by her son Liam's fight against cancer but appalled that treatment options are not readily available because of the lack of funding needed. She decided to organize the largest bake sale ever, containing 96,000 cookies that were sold in three weeks, totaling $400,000! Her attempt to raise needed funds for research to enhance treatment options turned into a worldwide organization. "Be a good cookie" and host a bake sale to raise money for research to aide therapy for childhood cancer. There are Girl Scout opportunities for troops to earn badges for this cause. She has also partnered with ASICS shoes to design a gold and black athletic shoe embossed with the pediatric ribbon that supports pediatric cancer research with every purchase.
www.cookiesforcancer.org

Songs of Love is an organization that creates a song by a talented musician in honor of your child. The musicians are very particular in what they write, focusing on the melody and lyrics using parent/family input. They create a magical song that can be cherished by your child forever, free of charge.
www.songsoflove.org

Beads of Courage program is affiliated with 90 children's hospitals around the world. The bead necklace acts as a visual representation for children to document, share and own their treatment journey. The program uses colorful glass beads to represent different procedures and events that a child endures during treatment, their courage and journey. To date, Paris has a total of 25 necklaces that embrace many different beads and represent her treatments and procedures.
www.beadsofcourage.org

Erin's Dream Lanyards created in honor of Erin Buenger, symbolize a dream for a cure. At only12 years old, Erin lobbied Congress and raised money to increase funding and research for childhood cancer. The money earned from her dream wands supports neuroblastoma research through the Children's Neuroblastoma Cancer Foundation. www.chooseaverb.blogspot.com

The Princess Alexa Organization sent Paris a box of dress-up clothes. Alexa had neuroblastoma and loved to dress up while in the hospital. Her motto is "happiness is healing."
Princess Alexa Foundation
P.O. Box 274
Keller, Texas 76244
www.princessalexafoundation.org

Brooke's Blossoms N Buddies is a nonprofit organization created by Brooke Hester; a 5 year old diagnosed with neuroblastoma, and her mother Jessica, who became dedicated to making bald a beauty statement by creating magnificent, extravagant headbands as for children who have lost their hair. She is dedicated to creating awareness and sends headbands to children all over the world. www.brookefightsback.org

The Andrew McDonough B+ Foundation honors the memory of Andrew's motto, "Do Good." The B+ program is dedicated to families across the United States and has helped families who are struggling emotionally or financially with critically ill children. www.bepositive.org

Purses with a Purpose was started by Diana Cofield. She creates handmade tote bags and was inspired by a friend of ours named Morgan, who was diagnosed with neuroblastoma, to create and donate pink camouflage cancer awareness totes to represent the battle that these children face on a daily basis. It is an honor that Paris has one as she continues her fight.

Look Good...Fell Better is a nationwide program through the American Cancer Society that teaches girls and women who are experiencing hair loss to cope with skin and hair changes using cosmetic and skin products donated through the cosmetic industry, providing consultations and free cosmetic kits.
1-800-395-LOOK
www.lookgoodfeelbetter.org

Wigs for Kids is a nonprofit organization founded by Jeffery Paul. He provides custom handmade human hair replacements for children under 18 who lose their hair due to medical conditions.
1-440-333-4433
Email: info@wigsforkids.org

Face-to-Face Fine Art Commemorative Expressions, Inc., was started by D. Anne Jones, who works from photographs to provide free portraits to individuals who have lost a loved one to a sudden or unexpected death. This nonprofit organization wishes to ease the suffering and aid in the grieving process by providing a portrait that will honor the deceased.
www.facetofacefineart.com

Communication Resources

Facebook Groups
Many social media Facebook groups have formed and act as an internet forum or discussion site where individuals affected by neuroblastoma can hold conversations, vent, post comments and/or concerns. These are closed groups; however members can be added via Facebook. A few are listed below.

- Neuroblastoma Support Group. You Are Not Alone, Ask Away.
- Families Against Neuroblastoma (Fundraising, Awareness, Networking)

- Neuroblastoma Survivors
- Angel on my Shoulder
- Parents Who Lost Children to Cancer
- Band of Parents has an Angel Support Group

Caring Bridge Site and Care Pages-
Imagine telling the same story over and over again. One may get exhausted. One of the best modes of communication is the Caring Bridge or Care Pages website created for families with children who have any type of medical diagnosis. These are free websites to use and maintain that allow families to blog about their experiences and journey with a loved one with a serious illness. People tend to use Caring Bridge as the main method of communication to update people on recent news rather than being bombarded by phone calls. Other popular modes of communication that are commonly used are personal websites, blogs, or social media networks.
www.caringbridge.org
www.carepages.org

It is often suggested to have a website or page to display via internet for your child to alleviate you from having to repeat the same story over and over again every time the phone rings. It's a very good idea, but as with everything, you must be cautious on what type of information you post. Sometimes parents choose to password protect their site. In turn this can limit access to friends and family who are genuinely concerned to receive updates about your child. Once you post information about your child and it is available for the world to see, you open access to anyone to view the site, unintentionally inviting predators to use your information for their personal gain.

If you're going to set up a personal website or Caring Bridge site, you should consider following simple privacy suggestions, such as not posting your personal home address, phone number, social security numbers, or bank account numbers. If you are traveling to another facility for treatment outside of your home state, don't post the dates that you will be leaving. I used to post my updates after we returned, speaking about them in the past tense.

Ensure that you know and trust the people who are raising funds for you. There are people who will take information from your site, hold fundraisers, and then never turn over the profits. I suggest you search for your child's name on occasion to be aware of what pops up on the internet. I personally searched my daughter's name and learned that many people had posted YouTube videos of her, have her on their site, and even have her on their networking sites, such as MySpace, Twitter, Instagram, or Facebook. These posted representations of my daughter are harmless and were posted to spread the word about neuroblastoma and to share experiences and stories.

Care Calendar and Take Them A Meal are free calendar tools that allow people to assist families with errands, child care and meal planning during stressful times. www.carecalendar.org www.takethemameal.com

Education Resources

The Great West Division of the American Cancer Society has established a Survivor College Scholarship program to ease the financial and emotional hardship associated with fighting cancer giving young cancer survivors the opportunity to pursue their post secondary education.

Appendix 3: Treatments

Every year in the United States, approximately 13,000 children and adolescents are diagnosed with cancer. Twenty-five percent of those diagnosed will not survive. The mind is a powerful thing. It can hold you back, but it can also move you forward. Sometimes decisions that are made are placed into the category of "this is not an I want to but an I have to."

Following standard induction chemotherapies, if more therapies are needed due to a relapse, children tend to become immune to certain chemotherapy drugs. The doctors, therefore, have to keep switching up combinations, which then causes them to be classified as experimental, investigational, or clinical trial. At times, the only effective treatment is experimental and clinical trials for recurring neuroblastoma. This means the drugs recommended do not have enough literature published to establish effectiveness, which then in turn do not qualify them to be approved by the FDA.

Currently, there is no cure for neuroblastoma, therefore clinical trials are deemed as the standard measure of care, and ultimately the only means of survival for these children. Insurance companies deny treatment based on the fact that it is not approved by the FDA. If treatment by insurance is denied, families are forced to either participate in experimental/investigational treatments at their own expense, go with another treatment plan that may not be as strongly recommended, or place their children on hospice. How can people in the insurance companies and the FDA live with themselves knowing that their denial has the potential to cause a death of a child?

Years ago the diagnosis of neuroblastoma was still present; however treatment options did not vary as much as they do today. Research and technology have come a long way. Ten years ago, children with neuroblastoma unfortunately didn't survive long enough to receive all of the treatment options that they do today. The disease was considered fatal. I can only hope and pray that my daughter is here long enough to see a cure discovered.

Treatment options change on a regular basis as advances are made. All studies are not open to all patients. Usually there is a set criteria that patients must meet to enroll in the study. The oncology team will be able to help navigate through the available trials and enrollment criteria. The website www.clinicaltrials.gov is a registry and database of publicly and privately supported clinical studies of human participants conducted around the world.

There are so many hospitals all over the world that deal with childhood cancer, so as a parent with a child who has cancer, how do you choose the best facility? Ralph and I were faced with difficult decisions like this on a regular basis. I constantly felt like a walking T-chart, analyzing the pros and cons of every possible treatment plan and situation presented to us. One decision that I am always conflicted with is do we give Paris medications and toxins that could possibly help her now but potentially hurt her in the future? The answer that Ralph and I have agreed upon is that we have to think about the present and do what's right at the particular moment, with Paris' quality of life as a determining factor.

Hospitals are very competitive and all have very different treatment plans. There are different options out there to treat neuroblastoma, and sometimes I wonder if I am doing the right thing. There are restrictions to the treatment plans, and it becomes very confusing. I have been fortunate that my home hospital has maintained a relationship with Memorial Sloan-Kettering, creating a team approach and collaborative efforts for the best interest of Paris.

As a parent of a child with cancer, specifically neuroblastoma, I wanted to locate the best possible care for my child, even if that meant I needed to travel to another country. If that's where the best was, then that's where I was destined to go.

It's extremely difficult to be treated somewhere for so long, build a rapport with the staff, establish a level of comfort, and then all of a sudden have cancer strike with a vengeance, without any warning. That very team that has been with you through thick and thin says, "I'm sorry, there is nothing else we can do. We have exhausted all of our treatment options." It's amazing that as a parent, the very next day you will research any treatment facility that has something to offer, jump on a flight, and start again with someone else just for that ray of hope.

I have heard so many families say time and time again, "I have never heard of that hospital facility or treatment protocol, plan, or trial." I want to inform parents that are new to the world of neuroblastoma about all of their options so they can make the best-educated decisions regarding their children.

When you become part of the cancer world, we as a group of parents know that there are specific hospitals where patients tend to travel to receive specialized care.

Memorial Sloan-Kettering in New York City: The doctors there are Dr. Nai Kong Cheung, Dr. Kushner, Dr. Modak, Dr. Kramer, Dr. Waldon, and Dr. LaQuaglia. This team has been recognized to have devised the best clinical trial treatments available. Dr. LaQuaglia is noted as the best surgeon in the field to remove masses that no other surgeon will consider removing.

The team puts a key focus on antibody treatment because antibodies do not damage DNA, and thus far there are no discovered late effects associated with antibody treatment compared to the standard measure of care. Antibodies are proteins that help the immune system recognize foreign substances by binding to them and marking them for removal. Neuroblastoma arises from normal tissue within the body; therefore the immune system tends not to recognize cancer cells as foreign bodies.

Sloan-Kettering offers a number of recognized treatments. Antibody 3F8 uses Rituxan to prevent HAMA. 3F8 is a monoclonal antibody that is injected into the bloodstream and travels into the body until it finds and attaches to a marker called GD2, which is present on neuroblastoma cells. Antibody 8H9 is a monoclonal antibody used as a treatment when neuroblastoma has metastasized to the brain. 8H9 is linked to radioactive iodine and infused directly into the cerebrospinal fluid. Prior to the 8H9 antibody, developed at Memorial Sloan-Kettering, no child survived once neuroblastoma entered the brain or spinal cord. A central nervous system (CNS) relapse was considered 100 percent fatal. Memorial Sloan-Kettering began using antibody 8H9 in 2003 in attempts to fight the disease in the CNS.

Turbo 3F8 is a $1.5 million project funded by Dena Sherwood, through Arms Wide Open, which won the Pepsi challenge grant of $250,000 to aid the trial. There are vials of humanized 3F8 antibodies that exist waiting for FDA approval. The theory is that you are inducing an antibody that the body will remember to create on its own to prevent the tumor from growing back.

The Protocol 05-075 clinical vaccination trial for one year is offered at Sloan-Kettering, where the child receives a total of seven shots. The first three are given during weeks 1, 2, and 3. It is then combined with a beta glucan supplement for two weeks on and two weeks off for a period of one year.

Sloan-Kettering reports that the success of bone marrow transplant is 20 percent, success of 3F8 is 40 percent, success of 3F8 with granulocyte-macrophage colony-stimulating factor (GM-CSF) is 60 percent, and the success of 8H9 is more than 80 percent.

Memorial Sloan-Kettering has a new clinical trial involving a weekly infusion of IMC-A12 Anti-IFG-I Receptor Monoclonal Antibody. IMC-A12 inhibits the action of protein needed for cell growth and may kill cancer cells.

It also has a stage 1 trial that uses Temsirolimus and Perifosine, which are drugs that cross the blood brain barrier and have shown to inhibit and kill cancer cells.

Children's Hospital of Philadelphia (CHOP): Dr. Maris (maris@email.chop.edu) and Dr. Mosse conducted the anaplastic lymphoma kinase (ALK) inhibitor trial. The team examines preserved neuroblastoma tumor samples to determine if the cells contain the inherited ALK gene mutation or the non-inherited form. The testing takes four weeks and is costly, and insurance may not cover it. CHOP has the internal capability to do genetic profiling to create a personalized therapy approach to neuroblastoma. The name of the proposal is Individualized Management of Pediatric Cancer-Neuroblastoma. The driver mutations of neuroblastoma have been identified in the lab, which allows the genetic profiling team to develop individual target therapy approaches. Another popular protocol, the Phase II trial of ABT751, ran from 2007 to 2009 at CHOP, however it is currently closed.

Cincinnati Children's Hospital ANBLO931 Chimeric Antibody 14.18 (CH 14.18) with GM-CSF: Cincinnati Children's Hospital has developed a new treatment using viral-based therapies that have linked using the herpes simplex virus to prevent the spread of neuroblastoma cells. The therapy causes them to self-destruct by using bovine herpes virus VP22.

UCSF San Francisco Medical Center: Dr. DuBois and Dr. Matthay focus on high-dose chemotherapy and stem cell transplant as the standard measure of care as well as the humanized antibody CH14.18.

The University of Texas MD Anderson: Dr. Zage and Dr. Reynolds (patrick.reynolds@ttuhsc.org) have used the recognized treatment ABT-751. Dr. Crystal Louis and Dr. Malcolm Brenner at Texas Children's Cancer Center for Cell and Gene Therapy (TXCCC) have conducted neuroblastoma trials for children with relapsed or refractory disease through the use of the Allogeneic Tumor Cell

Vaccination with oral metronomic Cytoxan trial and the ATOMIC trial.

University of Minnesota: This hospital focuses on the Seneca Valley Virus for neuroblastoma.

St. Jude in Memphis, Tennessee: This hospital focuses on the ANGI01 with Fariba Navid and the NB2005 trial. Memorial Sloan-Kettering is working in collaboration with St. Jude regarding the genome project. The purpose of this study is to determine the makeup of the tumor to help develop targeted treatments. Gene Arrays provides information regarding DNA, RNA, and more than 50,000 genes. The biologic information will be kept for future analysis. The cost to obtain the information is expensive, and most insurance companies do not cover it because it is seen as not medically necessary. You may be able to enroll in the procedure if there is a current study going on so you don't have to pay for it out of pocket. Gene Arrays could predict what types of chemotherapies the child may or may not respond to.

Van Andel Research Institute (VARI), Grand Rapids, MI.: Dr. Giselle Sholler and the VARI team focus on the Neuroblastoma and Medulloblastoma Translational Research Consortium (NMTRC) trial. Her direct email is giselle.sholler@helendevoschildrens.org. Another trial conducted in Michigan is TPI 287 & DMFO.

Dana Farber at the Children's Cancer Hospital of Boston, Mass.: Dr. Shamberger focuses on I-131 MIBG therapy and stem cell transplant. MIBG therapy is a radioactive drug delivered intravenously that travels to the tumor sites delivering radiation. MIBG is less toxic then chemotherapy and is considered standard measure of care for recurrent neuroblastoma patients in Europe and the United States.

Riley Children's Hospital in Indiana: Indiana's only comprehensive children's hospital, with pediatric specialists in every field of medicine and surgery, Riley provides clinical care and conducts research for children with cancer.

Ann & Robert H. Lurie Children's Hospital of Chicago, formerly Children's Memorial Hospital: Lurie is one of the top pediatric providers in the Midwest, treating children with the highest quality of care.

Children's Hospital Los Angeles: Dr. Araz Marachelian, Dr. Seegar, and Dr. Shimada focus on innovative neuroblastoma research.

Comer Children's Hospital at University of Chicago: Dr. Cohen; a highly respected expert in pediatric cancers, and team actively research aspects of neuroblastoma.

It is up to parents to search out and choose which facility and treatment options are best for newly diagnosed and/or relapsed neuroblastoma patients. You can only make the best-educated decision for your child with the information that is at hand at that particular time. As a parent you need to stay informed and never just agree with what is being presented. You need to ask questions and seek out all of the other treatment plans. Asking questions will allow you to rationalize and weigh all your options to make the best-educated decision regarding your child's treatment plan and be informed of the possible side effects that clinical trials and protocols may bring on later in life as a direct effect of the treatment. Knowing all of the information will help you make the best-educated decision regarding your child. The website www.clinicaltrials.gov provides parents with a list of open and available trials with the most recent developed treatment plans in which children can participate. It also allows parents to limit the search to relapse trials when applicable.

New Approaches to Neuroblastoma Therapy (NANT) is a group consisting of 13 universities and children's hospitals that design and implement Phase 1 and Phase 2 clinical trials that combine the use of various drugs. www.NANT.org

Cure Search for Children's Cancer (COG) is a children's oncology group that works together to pioneer treatments and cures. There are common trials, such as COG-ANBLO532-Phase 3 trial, human antibody Cixutumumab Phase 2 trial, COG-ADVL0821, COG-ANBL0032 trial and COG's Phase 3 trial 3891, which showed an 11 percent survival rate for patients who had transplant versus those who did not. These participants did not receive antibody treatment. www.curesearch.org Since 2009 Ch14.18, a monoclonal antibody designed to bind to neuroblastoma cells while stimulating the patient's immune system to kill cancer, has been standard care for high-risk neuroblastoma patients treated at COG.

According to COG and the American Cancer Society, the five-year survival rate refers to the percentage of patients who live at least five years after their cancer has been diagnosed. The national average survival rate for five years is 76.4 percent. That statistic sounds good, but it must be clarified for people outside of the cancer world because it does not mean overall survival. When Paris was diagnosed at 9 days old, that national statistic gave us 76.4 percent hope that she would survive for the next five years, placing her at 5 years old. Children diagnosed within the low-risk group have a five-year survival rate of 95 percent. Children diagnosed in the intermediate risk group have a five-year survival rate of 80 to 90 percent, and children in the high-risk group have a five-year survival rate of 30 to 50 percent. According to Memorial Sloan-Kettering, after considering all factors, Paris had a 30 to 50 percent chance of obtaining a five-year survival rate after her initial diagnoses. However, when she was diagnosed at 9 days old and then relapsed four more times, it significantly decreased her survival rate to less than 5 percent.

There are so many combinations of treatment plans offered to children with cancer all over the United States. The trick is finding the right fit for your child and feeling confident with the decision that you make. Whether it be chemotherapy, radiation, surgery, antibodies, vaccines, homeopathic therapies, or other clinical trials, they're all in attempts to find the golden ticket for your child. Until there is a cure, there is no right answer...only hope.

Through all of the treatments and all of the side effects, Paris was able to maintain a level of happiness that most people never reach. She overcame each challenge and faced it with so much courage and strength. Never once did she let this disease change her. She has a very determined personality, strong mindset, and is full of bravery. She has continued to be the most compassionate, helpful and considerate child toward others, even though the most horrific pain has been brought upon her.

Appendix 4: Tricks of the Trade

When I was first introduced to the cancer world, I felt alone and didn't know what to do. I wish that there was a 1-800 number or a guidebook readily available to me. When I looked on the internet regarding others and their experience with neuroblastoma, there wasn't much information available. I decided to incorporate this section because these are some of the things that I learned along the way.

Every time I snuggle with Paris, I get a passing thought that at that very same moment there is someone out there mentally, physically, or emotionally abusing their child. I can't sometimes move beyond the thought that people would go out of their way to abuse or neglect their children. At those moments, I can only squeeze Paris that much tighter and make sure that she feels nothing but love and affection all of the time, as her time here on Earth is not guaranteed and I want her to always enjoy every minute.

During Paris' treatment I felt like I had to clean all of the time. Your home will be consumed with hand sanitizer and anti-bacterial wipes in each room. Paris has not received transplant, however the hospital advised not to get any new pets, to replace toothbrushes at least once a week, to watch Paris' diet and limit the glucose, sugar, and sodium, to vacuum daily, to keep visitors away, to use paper towels instead of regular towels, to not use the fireplace, and to frequently clean out the vents. I used Clorox wipes to clean anything that would be frequently touched (doorknobs and railings) and everyone who entered wore masks.

Potassium Iodide Oral Solution (SSKI drops) are given to protect the thyroid before, during, and after MIBG scans. Patients receive seven drops over three days. They taste horrible alone, so parents tend to mix them to hide the taste. Paris was only an infant when we had to start SSKI drops, so it wasn't as easy as explaining it to her or rationalizing the reasons behind it. I mixed the seven drops with flattened sprite in a small cup and then pre-drew the mixture up to about 5 milliliters. I was careful not to add too much sprite in the event that Paris did not finish the mixture, and I would hold her down and shoot it into the corner of her mouth, back toward the throat without a problem. I learned very quickly to ensure that the sprite was not bubbly because Paris would cough and gag as I shot the syringe down her throat, causing her to throw up the entire dose of SSKI, which meant we had to re-dose. I also found it better to give her the drops right after she woke up from sedation, as she was still groggy and not yet awake, resisting her will to fight. Other parents say mixing it with drinks such as root beer, apple juice, or water worked for them. One parent said that dipping cookies into milk and then dropping the seven drops onto the cookie worked. Other parents have been able to slip the drops into their child's mouth them while they are sleeping and then they chase it with juice or water.

During treatment, many children lose a tremendous amount of weight, which can impact the scheduled radiation and chemotherapy treatments. Some helpful ways that I found to increase weight was to supplement with nutricia Duocal, which is a super soluble powdered energy source that contains carbohydrates and fats. It can be added to any liquid and moist food without altering the taste or texture. There is 41 percent fat and 59 percent carbohydrates per 100 grams. Visit www.nutricia.com for more information. We also supplemented TPN and lipids through Paris' Medi-port for supplemental nutrition. There is an extremely thick pudding supplement called Boost, which comes in strawberry, chocolate, and vanilla flavors. If your child is able to digest solid foods, you can cook with real butter and serve a diet rich in fatty foods.

Dieticians recommend drinking PediaSure for daily vitamins. Paris' dietician stated that one of the best ways to gain weight was to eat Haagen Daz vanilla ice cream, which contained 270 calories per ½ cup serving. According to dieticians, antioxidants and omega 3 fatty acids incorporated into meals may support your child's already compromised immune system by adding omega 3, vitamin D, calcium supplements, and an overall multivitamin. Some of the supplements recommended for long-term antioxidant support include green tea and soy protein.

People have used GLAD plastic wrap or press and seal wrap to cover central lines and Medi-ports to protect them from water. It works well during bath time – otherwise they can't take a bath for seven days! GLAD has developed a partnership with Cookies for Cancer to help raise awareness for childhood cancer.

It is recommended that children do not routinely receive Tylenol (Acetaminophen) with vaccinations because it lowers the antibodies. Asprin, Motrin, or Aleve are generally not used in pediatric cancer patients because they inhibit platelet function and may cause severe bleeding in a thrombocytopenic patient.

At Children's Memorial Hospital, Paris regularly obtained Fentynal as an anesthetic. At Memorial Sloan-Kettering, she was given Propofol, which is said to be the only anesthetic that has not yet been shown to depress the immune system. Young patients that receive this drug commonly refer to it as the "milky medicine." It's a thick, white drug, and honestly as soon as it enters into the blood stream, the child falls asleep. It happened to be the same sedation drug that Michael Jackson used, however his quantity of daily usage was over the recommended dose.

Appendix 5: Insurance

Approximately 46 children are diagnosed with cancer daily. Far too many are dying because there is currently not a cure for neuroblastoma. It is considered an "orphan disease" because pharmaceutical companies do not see the efforts as profitable, meaning they will not adopt the cause to find a cure. There are simply not enough children fighting neuroblastoma to attract the attention of profit-driven pharmaceutical companies. As a consequence, the mortality rate has remained at 85 percent for 30 years. Doctors are frantically trying to conduct research to fund and create treatments that are not FDA approved and considered experimental/investigational until a cure is found. Many nonprofit organizations and parent groups take matters into their own hands to raise money and awareness in various ways to aide in funds specifically for neuroblastoma research. Their goal is to "celebrate more birthdays than funerals."

The best treatment in the world is no good to you if you can't receive it or gain access to it. No one should die because they can't afford health care, and no one should go broke because they get sick.

Insurance companies determine what is experimental versus standard measure of care or medically necessary. If your child has been on a standard care/treatment plan and it is still not working, then it is often suggested by the oncology team that your child would need to be part of a clinical trial. Many, if not all, plan language refuses to approve experimental, clinical, or investigational treatments that are not FDA approved. Many times, treatment options are denied and left as the patient's financial responsibility. As a result of those denials, a parent can choose to do two things: nothing and accept the decision or write an appeal letter.

It's not like I want to put my child through these types of horrific treatments that have the potential to have long-term effects. We are told that the treatment may be the only way, and without it your child will die. The doctors are telling you, "We don't know if the medication will work, but we do know the side effects are most likely guaranteed." Do you take that risk? What would you do? How do you make a decision after hearing the worst? Would you accept the decision from people working from an insurance company that don't even know your children?

Writing an appeal is a plea to try and convince strangers to give a child permission to try a potential life-saving treatment that may be his/her only chance at survival. It is important to know the appeal process from your insurance company. Know beforehand what physicians and pharmacies participate in the insurance plans to avoid an out-of-network expense. Know the date on which it was denied and how long you have to appeal it. Be knowledgeable about how many levels of appeal there are, and consider that it may impact the schedule of treatment. Know who is on the appeal committee, who you can invite into the appeals process, such as a lawyer, and the credentials of the board making decisions on your proposal. It is important to have a copy of the denial in writing so that when you appeal it, you have proof of what they stated and the reasons why it was denied. Be prepared with a copy of the protocol, copy of your child's medical records, and a letter from your child's doctor regarding reasons for treatment. Be prepared to argue why your child's treatment is medically necessary. Remember, when it comes to your child, everything is medically necessary.

According to my insurance company I had 60 days to appeal, and I was allowed three appeals per service date. I think to myself, who has 60 days to gather, organize, and submit the needed documentation while their child is sick and going through the unimaginable?

I never thought that I'd be writing appeals to insurance companies to fight claims that have been denied medical coverage but have the potential to save my daughter's life. Writing the letters does not guarantee a change in decision. There have been times I have written letters and the decision of denial stood firm, while other times I have written letters and a portion or the entire amount that was originally denied was then fully covered.

My biggest appeal was when Paris' treatment plan was Temodar and Accutane. I contacted the insurance representative, and she informed me that she would send me a copy of the physician's review, but warned me about the 31 pages of graphic and disturbing information regarding Paris' long-term health and possible effects as well as the outcome for the overall disease. I thought to myself, I know that this disease is life threatening, how much more horrible can it get? I read the report. The physician reviewing the claim was very supportive of the trials and felt that they were essential in her care and treatment plan, but insurance felt differently.

Temodar is part of the alkylating agent family. When given or prescribed in isolation, it is covered under insurance. Accutane is a drug used to treat acne, which is also said to work effectively to treat high-risk neuroblastoma, however, it is not FDA approved for that use. Paris' treatment plan is 42 days of Temodar followed by a two-week break. After the break, she would be prescribed Accutane. The insurance company, however, would not approve Accutane because it was not FDA approved and therefore considered experimental. It also would not cover Temodar when given in combination with Accutane, as a combination therapy is considered as two experimental drugs.

Having a good insurance plan has allowed Paris to receive quality medical care in a timely fashion without a lot of difficulty. Families who have a child with neuroblastoma who are not U.S. citizens and want to seek treatments at specific U.S. hospitals are required to put down a cash deposit of $300,000 before the hospital will consider them as a potential patient.

When something is denied, it's inevitable that creditors and billing offices will begin to call to collect payment, and it's like they have been trained to make you feel horrible. There must be a class that they take before getting hired, instructing them on phrases to say to make you feel guilty about not being able to pay the outstanding balance that I intentionally didn't create. A friend shared with us that a representative said, "Ma'am, we performed a service, and when people provide a service, it needs to be paid for." It seems that they have forgotten the insurance has already paid 80 percent of the entire bill; shouldn't that suffice?

It's always been my general rule not to pay things right away – just be patient. Resubmit the claims and let the insurance company process them. If you pay them right away, you lose your chance to appeal to the insurance company or the provider. You can often write a hardship letter to the provider. This might state that due to the ongoing medical care needed, you will continue to acquire a high-dollar amount in claims and request to be considered for a hardship, with the hope that the claims will be reconsidered and/or reduced for claims that are usual and customary. Sometimes if you explain that you cannot pay the full amount, they may be able to work out a payment plan, discount the balance, or wipe out the bill completely. Charity Care is money stored for hospital-related services. Patients are encouraged to communicate with hospital's financial advisors if they anticipate difficulty paying for their portion of the hospital bill. Charity Care programs can provide discounts up to 100 percent of hospital charges to those who are financially eligible.

Payments get crossed in the mail, and it seems like a forever game of cat and mouse. It is always important to review your bills that you have paid to ensure that you're not sending a duplicate payment because the previous amount may still be listed on your ongoing medical bill. It is important for you to know if the out-of-network benefits are the same as the in-network benefits and what the out-of-pocket deductible is for each. It is also important to call the insurance to frequently ask if you've reached it yet. Most insurance plans cap their coverage at $1 million. As a parent of a child with neuroblastoma, you will reach that cap in approximately 18 months.

For organizational purposes, every time you get an explanation of benefits from your insurance company document it in a spreadsheet or keep a very detailed organized file system. It will ease a lot of confusion when you have to reference the bills, claims, and explanations of benefits. Document every time that you speak with a representative, recording the name or ID number of the person, date of call, and brief explanation of what was discussed.

President Barack Obama was elected as the 44th president of the United States on November 5, 2008. One of his main goals was to change America's health care. According to the U.S. Census Bureau in 2008, 46.3 Americans did not have health care. That amounts to 15.4 percent of the U.S. population of 311,609,227, as estimated in the 2010 Census. Obama's Health Care Reform began with the Patient Protection and Affordable Care Act (PPACA), which became law on March 23, 2010. There are many pros and cons to ObamaCare depending on who is viewing the list; however one of the main components of this law prohibits insurance companies from denying coverage and claims based on pre-existing conditions.

Appendix 6: Long-Term Effects and Prognosis

Three out of five children that have been diagnosed with neuroblastoma suffer from long-term effects. Beating cancer doesn't prepare you for life's future obstacles. Long-term side effects depend on the extent of the disease, size, type, and location of the tumor, the tumor's response to therapy, the age of your child, and new developments in treatment.

As a parent with a child with cancer, you begin to weigh what is really important. There are a million recognized side effects as a result to the numerous treatments trying to fight cancer, and honestly, there are probably a million more that are unrecognized that may present later in life. So you end up weighing your options. You end up doing what needs to be done at the time and then deal with what may come later. When my mind becomes consumed of all the possible outcomes of receiving treatment, I tend to always remember someone saying, "We don't know if the medication we are administrating will work. But we do know that the long-term side effects are most likely guaranteed." I take that with a grain of salt because even though the chances of side effects for all that our children endure are great, I have met many long-term survivors who have not experienced what was predicted.

Paris may never be a mother because of the excessive ongoing treatment and radiation that she has received. It most likely damaged her reproductive organs at a very young age. Paris tells me all of the time that when she grows up she wants to be a mommy. I think about the day that she wants to get married and anticipates having children of her own. I think about having to tell her that that may not be possible for her, having to possibly discuss other options, such as adoption. However there are survivors who are able to have children despite the toxic treatment they have endured. I hope someday she will be able to experience having children of her own and experience the unconditional love that I feel toward her.

When a child is given a transplant, there are significant risks such as transplant-veno-occlusive disease (VOD), which can lead to kidney and or liver failure. This also applies to high-dose chemo, with the goal of wiping out the child's entire immune system and bone marrow and then re-infusing stored stem cells to "re-seed" the marrow. I have heard that if your child is undergoing Melphalan; give them a popsicle, ice cubes, or something cold to hold in their mouth during the infusion. It has been said to reduce the severity of mouth sores that come as an aftermath of the drug.

High-frequency hearing loss tends to occur with the use of chemotherapy or after a transplant over two years but is not limited to long-term effects. Cisplatin and carboplatin tend to affect hearing loss. Children may experience other ototoxicities such as Amikacin, which is used for neutropenic fevers, and Lasix for ascites that they have received over time while battling the disease. Their hearing can be assessed and tested by an audiologist using an audiogram to measure hearing abilities. If hearing loss is determined, hearing aides are typically recommended, and when children turn 3 years old, they can be eligible for school-related programs and accommodations established through a 504 plan. If possible, the hearing aids should be water resistant. There are some brands that digitally transpose high-frequency sounds into low-frequency sounds. For younger children, it is often hard to look different from their peers. Children find comfort in the use of Tube Riders, which are kid-friendly accessories that slide onto the earpiece tube to decorate the hearing aid. Parents can create favorite Disney characters by purchasing Disney Loomz charms and creating the same affect. Some common and popular brands of hearing aids that children with neuroblastoma purchase are Nios Micro V by Phonak or Oticon M5s.

Wisconsin's 2009 Senate Bill 27 requires insurance companies to cover both hearing aids and cochlear implants, as well as tests associated, for any patient under 18 who is a resident of Wisconsin. In the past, many insurance companies did not cover the cost of hearing aids, requiring parents to pay the expenses out of pocket.

A drug called sodium thiosulfate (STS) is being tested in children to determine if hearing can be protected from Cisplatin. One study showed that it was able to protect mice from losing their hearing, but it also protected the tumor. Researchers changed the dose, and now they say they can protect hearing without reducing the efficacy of Cisplatin. Hearing loss can affect high-frequency sounds, but it can also affect the middle pitches. Eighty percent of high-risk neuroblastoma patients lose some of their hearing.

Due to receiving chemotherapy at a young age, many children experience dental challenges, including enamel issues, limited developed roots, absent roots, and cavities. A panorex x-ray can determine if the roots are absent or if there was any other possible dental concern that may arise from receiving chemotherapy. Dr. Cherry is a dentist that works with children with neuroblastoma at Memorial Sloan-Kettering. Dentists recommend brushing with Omni gel, which is an added protection for the teeth, after the regular brush and fluoride.

Paris has had severe diarrhea after radiation, chemotherapy, and some surgeries. It is caused by the inability of the intestines to absorb water, an over-reaction to muscle layer of the intestine or damage to the rapidly dividing cells that line the intestine so that they cannot perform the function of absorbing liquid. Medications can be prescribed to help control cramping and diarrhea, such as pediatric Imodium or lomotil. It can also be minimized by maintaining a diet of clear liquids: water, apple juice, Jell-O, clear broth, popsicles, and ginger ale. An ointment called Dr. Smiths can treat severe diaper rash. As the diarrhea improves, the diet should consist of low-fiber foods such as white rice, boiled chicken, and mashed potatoes and then include foods high in potassium, which is an important mineral lost during diarrhea. These include eggs, cottage cheese, bananas, pasta, toast, applesauce, and crackers.

There is a noted link in some patient cases between chemotherapy and cognitive deficits. "Chemo brain" is a recognized term used to describe patients or survivors who have experienced difficulty with brain function as a result of chemotherapy, radiation, or surgery treatment. This may include symptoms such as difficulty multitasking, taking longer to complete tasks, lower attention spans, remembering details, learning new skills, disorganization, and exhaustion. When speaking with parents who have older children, they have stated that their children with chemo brain have been mislabeled as having Attention Deficit Disorder (ADD)-like symptoms. We will have to keep a close eye on Paris as she enters school to see if this affects her.

Acid reflux has been reported as a common side effect after induction chemotherapy. Drugs commonly used are Omeprazole (Losec), sulcrafate, pantoprazole, Zantac (Ranitidine), or proton pump inhibitors (Prilosec). Esophaguard, which is the natural citrus extract hematuria-n-N-acetyl-glucosamine (NAG), is found at vitamin shops, and is recommended if one experiences acid reflux. Overeating, excess liquid intake, caffeine, chocolate, and mint should be avoided.

Children who have undergone chemotherapy may feel motion sickness. Motion sickness patches usually calm an upset stomach for a duration of five days for cancer patients after chemotherapy. The FDA approved the patch Sancuso, which releases granisetron to block serotonin receptors. It is also available to cancer patients in tablet, solution, or injection form; however seizures are a possible side effect from the patch.

Due to certain treatments, children may at times break out in viral infections, especially ones caused by the herpes simplex virus. Lysine is often used in treating the sores that commonly accompany the face or body of children after they undergo treatment.

I want Paris to be proud of her body and the marks that were left upon it. The trials and tribulations she has gone through helped her become the person she is today. I want to instill in Paris that her body is beautiful and just a physical part of her and that the appearance does not matter. It is important for her to understand that these countless marks and scars mean that she is alive, and she should be proud of the hard work that she has endured to be where she's at today. It's the soul that counts. It's how you present yourself as a person that truly matters in life.

A friend who had battled cancer and who is now an adult commented on the scars he sees when he looks in the mirror. He was almost bothered that they were there, as they were a daily reminder of what he went through.

I replied, "Remember, the scars are a daily representation of what you went through to be here today. They are a symbol of strength. Embrace them and be proud of your war wounds." I can only hope that Paris can be proud of her entire self and be proud of whom she is and what she went through and not let people's stares or possible comments affect her spirit.

I have personally met survivors who are now in their late 30s, 40s, and 50s. I wanted to acknowledge that some individuals I have met along the way have grown into adulthood after having neuroblastoma as either an infant or child. As a parent going through this with my daughter, I rarely heard the stories where children survived and lived on as healthy adults, having families of their own after being told a grim outcome and limited chance of survival. Hearing these stories and knowing that there are people out there who have experienced the same things as your child gave me a sense of hope.

Epilogue

Life is a journey filled with lessons, hardships, heartaches, joys, celebrations, and special moments that ultimately lead us to our destination, our purpose in life. Challenges that we face will test our courage, strengths, weaknesses, and faith. Along the way we may stumble upon obstacles that will come between the paths we are destined to take. In order to follow the right path, we must overcome them. And sometimes these obstacles are really a blessing in disguise, only we do not realize it at the time.

Along the journey we will be confronted with many situations, some with joy and some filled with extreme heartache. Simply put, our reaction to these situations determines the kind of outcome we experience through the rest of the journey. When things do not go our way, we have two choices. We can focus on the fact that things did not go how we had hoped or we can make the best out of the situation and know that they are setbacks and find the lessons learned. Time stops for no one, and if we allow ourselves to focus on the negative, we may miss out on some really amazing things that life has to offer.

We can't go back to the past, we can only go forward with the lessons we have learned and experiences we have gained. It is heartache and hardships that actually help make us stronger people in the end. It is often said what doesn't kill you will make you stronger. It all depends on how one defines the word strong. In this sense, stronger means looking back at the person you were and comparing it to the person you have become today. It also means looking deep into your soul and realizing that the person you are today could not exist if it were not for the things that happened in your past.

Everything in life that's worthwhile requires a risk. If you don't take risks, you can't reap the rewards. If there is a possibility, then there is hope. Paris has impacted many people and continues to impact many people near and far on a daily basis. When there's a downfall, there is always an upside waiting.

There is nothing I wouldn't do for Paris. Before I became pregnant, I said to myself I would do anything for her, not knowing what to expect and that my life would be such as this, just knowing that anything that she needed, I would provide for her. After being in this situation I would do anything for her, give her anything, buy her anything despite finances, sacrifice happiness for her, sacrifice my own health for her and even die for her if I had too. She is my life and the most important thing to me.

To this date Paris' scans indicate stable, meaning that there are questionable areas still present, but until they change in size, one will never know if it is disease or simply remaining scar tissue. We began long-term follow-up care for pediatric cancer survivors, where Dr. Sklar at Memorial Sloan-Kettering will monitor and manage Paris' health on a yearly basis. We are just riding the calm wave for now, which feels very good. At times my mind tends to forget about the nature of this beast, but then something always pulls me back. I have to remind myself I am not at leisure to do that, even though it feels like we are living the normal life.

Whether you are just beginning this horrific nightmare, currently fighting to survive it, going through a relapse and beginning the fight all over again, or grieving, we made all of our choices along the way for the same purpose, for our kids.

Where do we go from here? The answer is unknown. The answer will always be unknown for me. The quest for perfect is unobtainable. Perfect doesn't really exist. Not for me, not for anyone. Perfect is simply what you make of your situation at hand.

I hope this book has served as a reference to help other people going through similar situations. Please remember that your kids are brave warriors, and to accompany them, you must be strong, find support, and have faith and hope.

Glossary

Abnormal: Deviating from what is normal or usual, typically in a way that is undesirable

Absolute Neutrophil Count (ANC): An estimate of the number of infection-fighting neutrophils (white blood cells) in your blood

Accutane (Isotretinoin): A form of vitamin A and used to treat severe nodular acne

Anaplastic Lymphoma Receptor Tyrosine Kinase (ALK Gene): The alteration or defect in a normal gene called Anaplastic Lymphoma Kinase; ALK is the only gene in which mutations are known to cause ALK-related neuroblastoma susceptibility

Anesthesia: Artificially induced by the administration of gases or the injection of drugs before surgical operations causing total or partial loss of sensation

Antibody (Immunoglobulin): A large Y-shaped protein produced by B-cells that is used by the immune system to identify and neutralize foreign objects such as bacteria and viruses

Antibody 3F8: A mouse-derived monoclonal antibody; a murine IgG3 monoclonal antibody that binds to GD2

Antibody 8H9: Radio-labeled (liquid radiation) antibodies deliver radiation specifically to any neuroblastoma cells that remain after surgery, chemotherapy or radiation therapies for patients who have had relapses in the brain or central nervous system

Antigens: A toxin or other foreign substance that induces an immune response in the body, especially the production of antibodies

Antineoplastic: Inhibiting or preventing the growth and spread of tumors or malignant cells

Apgar Test: Developed in 1952 by Virginia Apgar, the test is given 1 minute after birth and again after 5 minutes to evaluate a baby's condition in the areas of appearance, pulse, grimace, activity/muscle tone and respiration and scored between 0 and 10

Arrhythmia: Problem with the rate or rhythm of the heartbeat

Ascites: The buildup of fluid between the lining of the abdomen and abdominal organs

Atrial Ectopic Beats (AEB): A condition of the upper heart chamber that occurs before it would be expected

Attention Deficit Hyperactivity Disorder Predominantly Inattentive (ADHD-PI): Characterized primarily by inattention, easy distractibility, disorganization, procrastination and forgetfulness

Audiogram: A hearing test that measures and records how a person can hear different sounds and frequencies

Bacteria: Found in all natural environments, some bacteria can cause diseases in humans

Bactrim (Co-Trimoxazole, Trimethoprim-Sulfa): An antibiotic that helps to prevent or treat a specific type of pneumonia

Bell's Palsy: Dysfunction of cranial nerve VII, the facial nerve, which results in an inability to control facial muscles on the affected side, which can cause a temporary facial paralysis

Benign: A tumor, growth or condition that is not cancerous, lacking the ability to invade neighboring tissue or metastasize

Biopsy: A medical test commonly performed by a surgeon involving sampling of cells or tissues for examination

Blood Transfusion: Process of receiving blood products into ones circulation intravenously

Bone Marrow: Soft tissue in the center of the bones, where blood cells are produced

Bone Marrow Aspirations: Small pieces of bone, marrow and fluid that are taken from the front and back of the pelvic bone

Bone Scans: A radioactive tracer called technetium99 is injected and travels to areas of the bone that are affected with neuroblastoma

Bradycardia: An abnormally slow heart rate

BRCA Gene: A tumor suppressor gene that when inherited in a mutated state is associated with the development of various cancers, especially breast and ovarian

Broviac Line/Catheters: A long, hollow tube made of soft rubber-like material called silicone, with an opening called a **lumen**

Cancer: Uncontrolled growth of abnormal cells within the body

Carboplatin (CBDCA): A chemotherapy drug used to treat ovarian, lung and other cancers

Carpal Tunnel Syndrome: Pressure on the median nerve, which is a nerve in the wrist that supplies feeling and movement to parts of the hand

Catecholamine: Substances within the body that derive from the amino acid tyrosine and act as hormones that can be measured;

hormones that are completely released are dopamine, spinephrine and norepinephrine

Central Line: A catheter laced in large veins that can be used to administer medication directly into the blood stream

Central Nervous System (CNS): Composed of the brain and spinal cord, it controls most functions of the body and mind

Cephalic presentation: A situation where the fetus is in a longitudinal lie and the head enters the pelvis first

Cerebellum: The region of the brain that plays an important role in motor control

Cerebrospinal Fluid: The fluid that circulates through the brain and spinal cord

Chemo Brain: A term used by cancer survivors to describe a change in memory, concentration, attention, as well as the ability to perform different mental tasks after the completion of chemotherapy treatment

Chemotherapy (Chemo): The use of medications or drugs either oral or intravenous to treat cancer.

Choroid plexus cyst (CPC): Are cysts that occur within choroid plexus of the brain. The brain contains ventricles with a spongy layer of cells and blood vessels called the choroid plexus. The choroid plexus has the important function of producing a fluid called the cerebrospinal fluid

Cisplatin: A platinum containing chemotherapy drug used to treat cancers.

Clinical Trials: A study involving the effectiveness and safety of medications or medical devices by monitoring the effects on large groups of people

Colony-Stimulating Factor (CSF): A man-made protein very similar to naturally produced proteins in the body that predominantly signals the production of white blood cells

Complete Blood Count (CBC): Blood test that measures the concentration of white blood cells, red blood cells and platelets in a cubic milliliter of blood

Computed Tomography (CT): An imaging method that uses x-ray to create pictures of cross-sections of the body detecting neuroblastoma in the chest, abdomen and/or pelvis; prior to the scan, the child must intake radio contrast to outline the intestine

Controlled Groups: A group of subjects closely resembling the treatment group in many variables but not receiving the active medication or factor under study

Cyclophosphamide (Cytoxan): A highly toxic immunosuppressive antineoplastic chemotherapy drug to treat cancer

Cyst: An abnormal membranous sac containing a gaseous, liquid or semisolid substance

Deoxyribonucleic Acid (DNA): A molecule that encodes the genetic instructions used in development and functioning of all known living organisms

Dexamethasone (Decadron): Corticosteroid that treats inflammation and many other medical problems

Diploid: Cells with the same amount of DNA as normal cells

Diprivan (Propofol): An anesthetic used to induce or maintain anesthesia during surgeries, tests or procedures

Dopamine: A simple organic chemical that treats circulation problems

Doxorubicin (Adriamycin) "Red Devil": An anti-cancer antineoplastic chemotherapy used to treat a wide variety of cancers

Echocardiogram (Echo): A test that uses sound waves to create a moving picture of the heart

Electrocardiogram (EKG): A scan to track heartbeats

Epidural: Used in childbirth to produce loss of sensation below the waist.

Etoposide (VP-16): A chemotherapy that destroys cancer cells by interfering with the cancer growth cycle

Event-Free Survival (EFS): A measure of the proportion of people who remain free of a particular complication of disease after treatment that is designed to prevent or delay that particular complication

Explanation of Benefits (EOB): A statement sent by a health insurance company to covered individuals explaining what medical treatments and/or services were paid for on their behalf

Family Medical Leave Act (FMLA): Entitles eligible employees of covered employers to take an unpaid, job-protected leave of absence for specified family and medical reasons with continuation of group health insurance coverage under the same terms and conditions as if the employee had not taken a leave

Focal Radiation (Stereotactic Radiation Therapy): A highly targeted way of delivering radiation to treat cancerous tumors

Food and Drug Administration (FDA): A federal agency in the Department of Health and Human Services established to evaluate, regulate and approve the release of new foods and health-related products

Ganglioneuroblastoma: A type of treated or mature neuroblastoma that develops from nerve cells and is surrounded by ganglion cells

Ganglioneuroma: A neuroma containing ganglion cells; a mature neuroblastoma that is not malignant

Gastroesophageal Acid Reflux (GERD): A condition where the stomach contents (food or liquid) leak backward from the stomach to the esophagus

GD2: A disialoganglioside expressed on tumors of neuroectodermal organ

Genes: A molecular unit of heredity of a living organism

Gestational Diabetes: High blood sugar that starts or is first diagnosed during pregnancy

Granulocyte Colony Stimulating Factor/Neupogen (G-CSF): A growth factor that stimulates the bone marrow to make white blood cells. G-CSF may be used before high-dose chemotherapy to stimulate the bone marrow to make more stem cells

Granulocyte Macrophage Colony-Stimulating Factor (GM-CSF): A type of protein (colony-stimulating factor) that increases the number and activity of neutrophils

H1N1 or Swine Flu: Virus that is a subtype of influenza A and was the most common cause of human influenza in 2009

Hemangioma: A benign vascular tumor that is a buildup of blood vessels in the skin and usually appears as a red birthmark

Hemidiaphragm: Half of the diaphragm, the muscle that separates the chest cavity from the abdomen and that serves as the main muscle of respiration

Hemoglobin (HGB): Protein carried by the red blood cells that picks up oxygen in the lungs and carries it to tissues within the body

Homovanillic Acid (HVA): A major catecholamine metabolite used as an agent to detect oxidative enzymes and is associated with dopamine levels in the brain

Human Anti-Mouse Antibodies (HAMA): Measures how strongly the body's immune system is reacting to 3F8.

Human Anti-Mouse Antibodies (HAMA) Positive: Term used when the patient has developed an immune response against neuroblastoma and can no longer receive antibody 3F8

Human Epidermal Growth Factor Receptor 2 (HER 2): A breast cancer that tests positive for a protein called HER2, which promotes the growth of cancer cells

Hydromorphone (Dilaudid): A narcotic pain reliever used to treat moderate to severe pain

Hydronephrosis: Condition where the kidney(s) become swollen or stretched as a result of a buildup of urine inside the kidney(s)

Hyperdiploid: Neuroblastoma cells with increased DNA

Immune System: The body's defense system against disease

Immunosuppressed System: The impaired ability of the immune system to fight infection or other diseases

Individual Education Plan (IEP): A legal document that guides the delivery of special education services and support services for students with disabilities

Induction Chemotherapy: The first stage of treatment where chemotherapy is used to reduce the number of cancer cells

Inferior Vena Cava (IVC): The large vein that carries deoxygenated blood from the lower half of the body into the right atrium of the heart

Inflammatory Bowel Disease (IBD): Chronic inflammation of all or part of your digestive tract

Influenza (Flu): An infection of the nose, throat and lungs

Insuflon Catheter: An indwelling soft plastic catheter placed just below the skin for frequent injections without the use of an actual needle sticking the child

Intensive Care Unit (ICU): A special department of the hospital where staff are highly trained to care for patients who rapidly deteriorate or who have recently had invasive surgery with high-risk complications

Intermediate Tumor: A tumor that contains benign and malignant cells

International Neuroblastoma Staging System (INSS): A system used by the cancer care team to determine the extent of the cancer; stage determines which risk group the child falls into, which in turn affects treatment options

Intrathecal: Refers to the fluid-filled spaces between the thin layers of the tissue that cover the brain and spinal cord, known as the cerebrospinal fluid

Intravenous (IV): Refers to giving medications or fluids through a needle or tube inserted into a vein

Invasive Ductal Carcinoma (IDC): The most common form of breast cancer that begins growing in the duct and invades the fatty tissue of the breast outside of the duct

Irinotecan: A chemotherapy drug extracted from the camptotheca acuminate, a plant that grows in Asia and kills cancer cells by interfering with the enzyme topoisomerase 1

Leptomeningeal (Thin Meninges): A term used to refer to the pia mater and arachnoid mater, two membranes that surround the brain and the spinal cord

Leukemia: A form of cancer that affects the blood-forming cells of the bone marrow

Leukine (Sargramostim): Used to help increase the number and function of white blood cells after bone marrow transplant, before or after stem cell transplant, and following chemotherapy treatment

Leukocytes (White Blood Cells): Cells of the immune system used to fight infections and other foreign substances

Lidocaine/Prilocaine (Emla Cream): Applied to the skin to cause numbness or loss of feeling before a certain medical procedure

Lipids (Fats): Any group of organic compounds that are fatty acids

Lymph Node: Small bean-shaped glands throughout the body, they can swell in one location when a problem such as injury, infection or tumor develops

Lymphatic System: Carries fluid, nutrients and waste materials between the body tissues and the bloodstream

Magnetic Resonance Imaging (MRI): A scan that uses magnetic fields and pulses of radio wave energy to create pictures of organs and structures inside the body, specifically the brain and spinal cord

Malignant: A cancerous tumor that invades normal tissue

Mammogram: An x-ray picture of the breast(s)

Mammography: The process of using low energy x-rays to examine the human breast(s); it is used as a diagnostic and screening tool

Medically Necessary: Referring to a covered service or treatment that is absolutely necessary to protect and enhance the health status of a patient

Medi-port (Portacath): A small medical appliance that is installed beneath the skin

Meninges: The system of membranes that envelop the central nervous system

Metastasize: To grow or spread from one part of the body to another

Metaiodobenzylguanidine (MIBG) Injection (Iodine-131): Radioisotope that is injected into a vein to locate or confirm the presence of tumors of the nervous system

Metaiodobenzylguanidine (MIBG) Scan: A nuclear imaging test that uses a radioactive substance (radioisotope tracer) to find or confirm the presence of tumors within the body

MIBG scan: Radioactive meta-iodobenzylguanidine (MIBG), which attaches to neuroblastoma cells after it has been injected into the blood stream and lights the area up; older children do not need to be sedated during this scan because they can understand that they need to lay still; in these cases, families may be in the room during the scan

Monocytes: White blood cells that are produced in the bone marrow and are part of the immune system of vertebrates

Morphine: A drug that treats moderate to serve pain

Mucositis: Painful inflammation of the mucous membranes lining the digestive tract; usually an adverse effect from chemotherapy

Mutations: A change in the DNA sequence

MYCN: A protein and member of the MYC family of proto-oncogenes; it is able to simultaneously control how cells grow and how they die

N-Myc: Proto-oncogene protein, or N-Myc or basic helix-loop-helix protein 37, is a protein that in humans is encoded by the MYCN gene and plays a role in the development of human tumors

N-Myc Gene Amplification (NMA): An overexpression of the N-Myc gene can be associated with a variety of tumors, frequently neuroblastoma; in cancerous cells, MYCN amplification has the unfortunate result of putting too much emphasis on cellular growth and not enough weight on cellular death, causing rapid tumor progression

N-Myc Non-Amplified: The absence of N-Myc amplification

Naloxone Chloride (Narcan): An opiate receptor that reverses the effects of certain types of medications; it is often used in life-threatening situations

Narcotics: A drug that, in moderate doses, dulls the senses, relieves pain and induces profound sleep, but in excessive doses can cause coma or convulsions

Nasogastric Intubation Tube (NG): Specialized tube that carries food and medicine to the stomach through the nose

Natural Killer Cells (NK): A lymphocyte able to bind to certain tumor cells and virus-infected cells without the stimulation of antigens and kills them

Neoplasm: An abnormal mass of tissue, which maybe solid or fluid filled, that results when cells divide more than they should or do not die when they should

Neuroblastoma (NB): A malignant (cancerous) tumor that develops from nerve tissue; it is the most common extracranial solid cancer in childhood and the most common cancer in infancy.

Neuroma: The growth or tumor of nerve tissue that tend to be benign

Neurons: An electrically excitable cell that processes and transmits information through electrical and chemical signals

Neutropenia: A condition that occurs when the number of neutrophils in the body is extremely low

Neutrophils (White Blood Cells): An immune cell that helps fight bacterial and fungal infections within the body

No Evidence of Disease (NED): A term to indicate that the signs and symptoms are no longer present; however, it is possible that cells may continue to exist in the body at a level that testing methods cannot detect

***Nil Per Os*/Nothing by Mouth (NPO):** A medical instruction that prohibits the intake of food or fluids

Nystatin: A polyene antifungal medication to treat infections caused by fungus

Obsessive Compulsive Disorder (OCD): An anxiety disorder in which people have repeated or unwanted thoughts, feelings, ideas, sensations, (obsessions) or behaviors that make them feel driven to do something (compulsions)

Ommaya Reservoir: A soft plastic dome connected to a catheter that is placed into a cavity of the brain

Oncogene: A gene that normally directs cell growth, however if altered can promote or allow uncontrolled growth of cancer

Oncologist: A specialist in oncology

Oncology: The study and treatment of tumors

Ondansetron (Zofran): A medicine to help prevent nausea and vomiting caused by cancer medicines

Operating Room (OR): A room in a hospital specially equipped for surgical operations

Oral Candidiasis (Thrush): An infection of the mucus membrane lining of the mouth or tongue caused by candida fungus (yeast)

Orthopedist: A specialist in correcting deformities of the skeletal system, especially in children

Ototoxicity: Damage to the hearing or balance functions of the ear by drugs or chemicals

Paclitaxel (Taxol): An antineoplastic agent (cancer medicine) used to treat the breast, lung and ovarian cancer

Parietal Lobe: Located above the occipital lobe and behind the frontal lobe, it integrates sensory information from different modalities, particularly spatial sense and navigation

Pathology: The precise study and diagnosis of a disease through examination of organs, tissue, bodily fluids and whole bodies (autopsies)

Pediatric Observation Unit (POU): Used to provide medical evaluation and or management for health-related conditions in children

Pentamidine: An antimicrobial medication given to prevent pneumocystis carinii pneumonia (PCP); a very serious type of pneumonia

Physical Therapy (PT): The treatment of physical dysfunction or injury by the use of therapeutic exercise intended to restore normal function or development

Platelets (Thrombocytes): Small blood components that help the clotting process by sticking to the lining of blood vessels

Pleural Effusion: The buildup of fluid between the layers of tissue that line the lungs and chest cavity

Ploidy: Number of set chromosomes in a biological cell
Pneumonia: Lung inflammation caused by bacterial or viral infection

Positron Emission Tomography Scan (PET): An imagining test that uses a radioactive substance called a tracer to show how organs and tissue are working and to look for disease in the body

Post-Traumatic Stress Disorder (PTSD): A type of anxiety disorder that can occur after you have gone through an extreme emotional trauma

Potassium Iodide Oral Solution (SSKI): A white, crystalline, water-soluble compound having a bitter saline taste used in medicine as an expectorant and to prevent or treat thyroid conditions

Pre-Existing Condition: A health condition that exists before someone applies for or enrolls in a new health insurance policy

Premature Atrial Contractions (PAC): One type of premature heartbeat, irregular heartbeat or benign arrhythmia

Progression-Free Survival: Refers to the interval from the date of diagnosis to the date of first documented disease progression or relapse

Proto-Oncogene: A normal gene that has the potential to become cancer because of mutations or some type of increased expression (expression is how information from a gene is utilized to create another genetic product)

Radiation: The process in which energy is emitted as particles or waves

Recurrent: Term used when a cancer returns to where it first started, another part of the body or to an area that has been previously treated

Response to Intervention (RTI): A method of academic intervention used in the United States to provide early, systematic assistance to children who have difficulty learning

Rituximab (Rituxan): A monoclonal antibody used to treat cancer

Sedated: To become calm or to put to sleep by administering a sedative drug

Septicemia: Bacteria in the blood

Septum: Dividing wall or partition of two things

Sodium Thiosulfate (STS): Colorless crystalline compound produced chiefly from liquid waste products of sodium sulfide or sulfur dye manufacture

SorbaView: Transparent film dressing that allows for a seven-day wear time

Stem Cells: Undifferentiated cells of a multicellular organism found in the human body that have the potential to develop into many different cell types and carry out different functions

T-Cells: Type of leukocyte (white blood cell) that orchestrates the immune system's response to infected or malignant cells

Tegaderm: A thin polyurethane membrane coated with a layer of adhesive used to cover and protect wounds

Temozolomide (Temodar): Belongs to the general group of medicines known as antineoplastics; a chemotherapy drug used to treat specific types of cancer of the brain

Thoracic Spine: The upper and middle back, it is made up of 12 vertebrae labeled T1 to T12

Thoraco Lumbo Sacral Orthosis (TLSO): A brace that comes in many designs and is used to immobilize the spine after a spinal surgery or injury

Thrombocytopenia: Low platelet count

Thrombosis: The formation of a blood clot inside a blood vessel obstructing the flow of blood through the circulatory system

Topoisomerase 1: Helps DNA unwind so that cells can reproduce

Total Parenteral Nutrition (TPN): A way of supplying all of the nutritional needs of the body by bypassing the digestive system and dripping nutrient solution directly into a vein

Transplant: To move or transfer something to another place

Tumor: An abnormal growth of body tissue

Ultrasound: Involves the use of high-frequency sound waves to create images of organs and systems within the body

Usual and Customary: The amount charged by a specific doctor that is considered the typical amount in the area that other doctors are charging

Vanillylmandelic Acid (VMA): A metabolic byproduct of norepinephrine and epinephrine used to detect neuroblastoma; VMA is elevated in the urine of patients with tumors that secrete catecholamines

Vascular Access Team (VAT): Individuals who are highly trained with starting an IV in the vein reducing the number of needle sticks patients have to endure

Veno-Occlusive Disease (VOD): Condition where some of the small veins in the liver are obstructed

Wilms Tumor: A rare type of kidney cancer that affects newborns and very young children

X-Ray: Electromagnetic radiation of short wavelength produced when high-speed electrons strike a solid target

CPSIA information can be obtained at www.ICGtesting.com
Printed in the USA
LVOW06s0743060614

388784LV00002B/222/P

9 781626 469730